Theophrastou Tou Eresiou Peri Ton Lithon Biblion. Theophrastus's History of Stones. With An English Version, and Critical and Philosophical Notes, Including The Modern History of The Gems

Theophrastus

Theophrastou tou Eresiou peri ton lithon biblion. Theophrastus's history of stones. With an English version, and critical and philosophical notes, including the modern history of the gems, &c. described by that author, ... By John Hill. To which are added
Theophrastus
ESTCID: T085893
Reproduction from British Library
The first seven words of the title transliterated from the Greek. With a list of subscribers. Parallel English and Greek text, with notes and additions in English.
London : printed for C. Davis, 1746.
xxiii,[1],211,[1]p. ; 8°

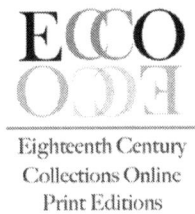

Eighteenth Century
Collections Online
Print Editions

Gale ECCO Print Editions

Relive history with *Eighteenth Century Collections Online*, now available in print for the independent historian and collector. This series includes the most significant English-language and foreign-language works printed in Great Britain during the eighteenth century, and is organized in seven different subject areas including literature and language; medicine, science, and technology; and religion and philosophy. The collection also includes thousands of important works from the Americas.

The eighteenth century has been called "The Age of Enlightenment." It was a period of rapid advance in print culture and publishing, in world exploration, and in the rapid growth of science and technology – all of which had a profound impact on the political and cultural landscape. At the end of the century the American Revolution, French Revolution and Industrial Revolution, perhaps three of the most significant events in modern history, set in motion developments that eventually dominated world political, economic, and social life.

In a groundbreaking effort, Gale initiated a revolution of its own: digitization of epic proportions to preserve these invaluable works in the largest online archive of its kind. Contributions from major world libraries constitute over 175,000 original printed works. Scanned images of the actual pages, rather than transcriptions, recreate the works ***as they first appeared.***

Now for the first time, these high-quality digital scans of original works are available via print-on-demand, making them readily accessible to libraries, students, independent scholars, and readers of all ages.

For our initial release we have created seven robust collections to form one the world's most comprehensive catalogs of 18th century works.

Initial Gale ECCO Print Editions collections include:

> ***History and Geography***
> Rich in titles on English life and social history, this collection spans the world as it was known to eighteenth-century historians and explorers. Titles include a wealth of travel accounts and diaries, histories of nations from throughout the world, and maps and charts of a world that was still being discovered. Students of the War of American Independence will find fascinating accounts from the British side of conflict.

Social Science
Delve into what it was like to live during the eighteenth century by reading the first-hand accounts of everyday people, including city dwellers and farmers, businessmen and bankers, artisans and merchants, artists and their patrons, politicians and their constituents. Original texts make the American, French, and Industrial revolutions vividly contemporary.

Medicine, Science and Technology
Medical theory and practice of the 1700s developed rapidly, as is evidenced by the extensive collection, which includes descriptions of diseases, their conditions, and treatments. Books on science and technology, agriculture, military technology, natural philosophy, even cookbooks, are all contained here.

Literature and Language
Western literary study flows out of eighteenth-century works by Alexander Pope, Daniel Defoe, Henry Fielding, Frances Burney, Denis Diderot, Johann Gottfried Herder, Johann Wolfgang von Goethe, and others. Experience the birth of the modern novel, or compare the development of language using dictionaries and grammar discourses.

Religion and Philosophy
The Age of Enlightenment profoundly enriched religious and philosophical understanding and continues to influence present-day thinking. Works collected here include masterpieces by David Hume, Immanuel Kant, and Jean-Jacques Rousseau, as well as religious sermons and moral debates on the issues of the day, such as the slave trade. The Age of Reason saw conflict between Protestantism and Catholicism transformed into one between faith and logic -- a debate that continues in the twenty-first century.

Law and Reference
This collection reveals the history of English common law and Empire law in a vastly changing world of British expansion. Dominating the legal field is the *Commentaries of the Law of England* by Sir William Blackstone, which first appeared in 1765. Reference works such as almanacs and catalogues continue to educate us by revealing the day-to-day workings of society.

Fine Arts
The eighteenth-century fascination with Greek and Roman antiquity followed the systematic excavation of the ruins at Pompeii and Herculaneum in southern Italy; and after 1750 a neoclassical style dominated all artistic fields. The titles here trace developments in mostly English-language works on painting, sculpture, architecture, music, theater, and other disciplines. Instructional works on musical instruments, catalogs of art objects, comic operas, and more are also included.

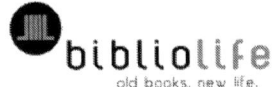

The BiblioLife Network

This project was made possible in part by the BiblioLife Network (BLN), a project aimed at addressing some of the huge challenges facing book preservationists around the world. The BLN includes libraries, library networks, archives, subject matter experts, online communities and library service providers. We believe every book ever published should be available as a high-quality print reproduction; printed on-demand anywhere in the world. This insures the ongoing accessibility of the content and helps generate sustainable revenue for the libraries and organizations that work to preserve these important materials.

The following book is in the "public domain" and represents an authentic reproduction of the text as printed by the original publisher. While we have attempted to accurately maintain the integrity of the original work, there are sometimes problems with the original work or the micro-film from which the books were digitized. This can result in minor errors in reproduction. Possible imperfections include missing and blurred pages, poor pictures, markings and other reproduction issues beyond our control. Because this work is culturally important, we have made it available as part of our commitment to protecting, preserving, and promoting the world's literature.

GUIDE TO FOLD-OUTS MAPS and OVERSIZED IMAGES

The book you are reading was digitized from microfilm captured over the past thirty to forty years. Years after the creation of the original microfilm, the book was converted to digital files and made available in an online database.

In an online database, page images do not need to conform to the size restrictions found in a printed book. When converting these images back into a printed bound book, the page sizes are standardized in ways that maintain the detail of the original. For large images, such as fold-out maps, the original page image is split into two or more pages

Guidelines used to determine how to split the page image follows:

• Some images are split vertically; large images require vertical and horizontal splits.
• For horizontal splits, the content is split left to right.
• For vertical splits, the content is split from top to bottom.
• For both vertical and horizontal splits, the image is processed from top left to bottom right.

ΘΕΟΦΡΑΣΤΟΥ τȣ ΕΡΕΣΙΟΥ

ΠΕΡΙ ΤΩΝ

Λ Ι Θ Ω ‘ Ν

ΒΙΒΛΙΟΝ.

THEOPHRASTUS's
History of STONES.

With an ENGLISH VERSION,

AND

CRITICAL and PHILOSOPHICAL NOTES,

Including the Modern History of the GEMS, &c. described by that Author, and of many other of the Native FOSSILS.

By *JOHN HILL.*

To which are added,

TWO LETTERS:

One to Dr JAMES PARSONS, F.R.S.
On the Colours of the *Sapphire* and *Turquoise*.

AND THE OTHER,

To MARTIN FOLKES, Esq; Doctor of Laws, and PRESIDENT of the ROYAL SOCIETY;

Upon the Effects of different Menstruums on *Copper*.

Both tending to illustrate the Doctrine of the GEMS being coloured by *Metalline Particles*.

LONDON,
Printed for C DAVIS, against *Grays-Inn* in *Holborn*,
Printer to the ROYAL SOCIETY.
MDCCXLVI

TO

HIS GRACE

CHARLES

Duke of RICHMOND, LENNOX, and AUBIGNY,

Earl of MARCH and DARNLEY,

Baron of SETTRINGTON and TORBOLTON,

One of the Lords of His MAJESTY's most Honourable Privy Council,

Master of the Horse to His Majesty,

LIEUTENANT-GENERAL,

AND

Knight of the Most Noble Order of the Garter.

MY LORD,

I Do myself the Honour of laying at your Grace's Feet, an Attempt to contribute something to the Study of the FOSSILE Kingdom, in an Ex-

A 2

planation of what one of the oldest Authors upon that Subject has left us, as every Part of polite Learning, and particularly what regards NATURAL HISTORY, has a kind of Claim, from the Honour of your Grace's Example, to your Grace's Patronage and Protection.

The Honour and Advantages that BOTANY, in particular, has received from your Grace's Regard, are strongly and in lasting Colours painted in those Gardens, where your Grace has so adapted the Soil and Situation, to Plants and Trees naturally the Product of the most distant Regions; that an Inhabitant of the Western World, entering the *American* Grove at GOODWOOD, would be astonished to see himself, as it were in a Moment, transported to his own Climate; nothing there striking his Eyes but the beautiful Productions of the Vegetable World in his own native Soil.

The Animal Kingdom is no less illustrated, in the noble Collection your Grace has made of the more wonderful Species of it; and particularly of the dreadful Beauties of the Serpent kind, Natives of warmer Climates: and which, to the Happiness of this Island, are here unknown unless in such Repositories; where their varied Paintings are not less pleasing, than their Presence, while living, is terrible.

Nor have the Curiosities of the Fossile World been denied a Place among the other many and wonderful Productions of Nature honoured with your Grace's Observation. But such is the Misfortune attending this Part of Natural Knowledge, that the Objects it offers, though not less beautiful, are yet less obvious to the Researches of even the most inquisitive Part of Mankind: A spreading Tree, an elegantly flowering Plant, or an extraordinary Animal, are Objects which directly meet the Eyes, and can hardly escape Observation; while Rocks of Gold and Masses of Gems, or what to a philosophic Eye is yet more admirable, the Parts of Plants or Animals, immersed in Stone, or buried under immense Quantities of Earth, are not to be found without searching for them at vast Depths within the Bosom of the Earth, where Nature first formed, or the Universal Deluge, or some other dreadful Catastrophe, has buried them, never by any natural Means to appear again.

This, my Lord, is one of the Discouragements under which this Study labours, and which has deterred Numbers of the Curious from entering upon it. If what I have here endeavoured to set in a new Light, may incite others to enquire into this Branch of Natural Knowledge, and to overlook these Difficulties, I shall have my full Reward.

Your Grace's Goodness will, I hope, pardon me that I cannot conclude this Address, without begging your leave *publickly* to express my great Obligations to Your GRACE on this Occasion, and acknowledging, with the warmest and sincerest Overflowings of a Heart full of Gratitude, that to your Grace alone, as the first Spring, is owing both this, and whatever else I may hereafter offer, since from your Grace's Goodness I have Leisure to prosecute these Studies: and that I must ever be, with the greatest Respect,

MY LORD,

Your GRACE's *most Obedient,*

And most Devoted Servant,

JOHN HILL.

A LIST OF THE SUBSCRIBERS.

THE Reverend Mr. Bryan Alliot.
Mr. Joseph Ames, *F. R. S.*
The Reverend Dr Angier.
Thomas Apreece, *Esq;*
Mrs D Apreece.
Mr. William Arderon, *F. R. S*

Lovewell Badcock, *Esq;*
Henry Baker, *Esq, F. R. S.*
Charles Balguy, *M D.*
Mr. George Barnard.
Mr. John Blackstone.
The Reverend Mr. John Branfoot.
Dr Brocklesby.

The Right Honourable the Countess of Chesterfield.
Mr. Mark Catesby, *F R S*
Samuel Clarke, *Esq, F. R. S.*

Dr. Mitchell.
Mr. Murray, *Surgeon.*

Mr. Turberville Needham.
Mr. James Nelson.
The Reverend Dr. Neve.
The Reverend Mr. Timothy Neve.

George Ogle, *Esq;*

James Parsons, *M. D. F. R. S. Three Books.*
Mr. Pierce, *Surgeon*
Mr. W. Potter, *Surgeon.*

Richard Richardson, *Esq;*
Benjamin Russell, *jun. Esq.*

The Honourable Charles Stanhope, *Esq,*
Dr. Peter Shaw.
Mr. Timothy Sheldrake, *Truss-maker.*
Mr. James Sherwood, *Surgeon*
Sir Hans Sloane, *Bart. M. D. F. R. S.*
Daniel Smyth, *Esq,*
The Gentlemens Society at Spalding.
Mr. William Strong.

The Right Honourable the Lord Viscount Tyrconnel.
The Reverend Mr. Talbot.
Mr. Isaac Terry.
The Reverend Mr. Tyson.

His Excellency Baron Waſſenaer.
Mr. William Watſon.
Mr. James Watſon.
Dr. Watſon
Dr. Wallis
Matthew Wildbore, *Eſq*,
Mr. George Wirgman.

Dr. Mitchell.
Mr. Murray, *Surgeon.*

Mr Turberville Needham.
Mr. James Nelson.
The Reverend Dr. Neve.
The Reverend Mr Timothy Neve.

George Ogle, *Esq*;

James Parsons, *M D. F. R. S. Three Books.*
Mr. Pierce, *Surgeon*
Mr. W. Potter, *Surgeon.*

Richard Richardson, *Esq*;
Benjamin Russell, *jun. Esq.*

The Honourable Charles Stanhope, *Esq,*
Dr. Peter Shaw.
Mr. Timothy Sheldrake, *Truss-maker.*
Mr. James Sherwood, *Surgeon*
Sir Hans Sloane, *Bart. M. D. F. R. S*
Daniel Smyth, *Esq*;
The Gentlemens Society at Spalding
Mr. William Strong.

The Right Honourable the Lord Viscount Tyrconnel.
The Reverend Mr. Talbot.
Mr. Isaac Terry
The Reverend Mr. Tyson.

His Excellency Baron Waſſenaer.
Mr William Watſon.
Mr. James Watſon.
Dr Watſon
Dr. Wallis.
Matthew Wildbore, *Eſq*,
Mr. George Wirgman.

THE
PREFACE.

THE many References to THEOPHRA-STUS, and the Quotations from him, so frequent in the Works of all the later Writers of Fossils, would make one believe, at first sight, that nothing was more universally known, or perfectly understood, than the Treatise before us: But when we come to enquire more strictly into the Truth, and examine with our own Eyes what it really is that he has left us, we shall find that though no Author is so often quoted, no Author is so little understood, or, indeed, has been so little read; those who are so free with his Name, having given themselves, generally, very little Trouble about his Works, and only taken upon trust from one another, what we shall in most Cases find, on a strict Enquiry, to have been originally quoted from him by *Pliny*, and as to that Author, whoever is acquainted with the Works of the more antient Writers, must know, that however much Praise he may deserve for that Treasure of Knowledge, he has, with almost infinite Pains, collected and handed down to us, yet he is very little to be depended on for the Correctness of his Quotations.

But it is no Wonder that the genuine Work of this Author on the Subject of Fossils, should have been so long and so much neglected to be read, since whoever shall take up even the best Editions of it we have at present, will find enough in every Page to dishearten him from making any farther Progress in it. The numerous Defects, *Lacunæ*, where whole Words, Parts of Words, and in some Places even many Words together are wanting; and the many Sentences, either by the careful Preservation of old Errors, or the injudicious Corrections of the Editors, rendered perfectly unintelligible, will soon shew, that it is a Work not to be read to any Advantage, without a more than ordinary Attention, a Knowledge of the Subject, and a continual Consultation of other of the Antients. Nor can it, indeed, be wondered at, that an Author who wrote more than Two thousand Years ago, and on a Subject so little understood, should be liable to numerous Errors in printing, which few of his Editors would have Capacity or Industry to set right.

In such Condition has this Treatise hitherto lain, full of excellent Matter, but rendered, in this Manner, almost unintelligible. The Author is remarkable for using very few Words; and where it was so common a thing, to find some of those few absolutely wanting, it seemed no easy Task rightly to understand him. On this Occasion, as also in regard to the Errors, so frequent and perplexing, I have been at the pains of consulting the rest of the Antients, in order to find what it was most likely he should say, by what they have said on the same Occasion. In these Undertakings, *Pliny* also, where he could be depended on, has been of singular Service, a Passage from him, frequently a literal Translation of this Author, shewing evidently how he had read the Original, who had the Advantage of seeing it, if not absolutely in its native Purity, yet at least before the Rise of many of the Errors that have made it much more unintelligible to us. This, and examining his Words by, and comparing them with the Substance he is describing, in such Cases where we are so happy to have the Substance yet in Use, are the two great Methods I have taken to understand him, and the last of them I have had the Happiness of more frequent Opportunities of referring

ring to than another Person naturally would have had, having been many Years making Collections for a History of the Medicinal Earths; and, on that Occasion, procuring Specimens of them, and of other Fossils, from various Parts of the World, and often from the very Places he is describing the Body he mentions to be produced in.

Where these Methods have not proved sufficient, I have had Recourse to the Critics; and as Reason, and either of the before named Assistances directed, have adopted the Opinions, sometimes of one, and sometimes of another. *De Laet* I have often had Occasion to name, for the Helps I have received from him; but, above all others, I have been most obliged to the excellent *Salmasius*: And notwithstanding that I have sometimes found it necessary to dissent from, and even censure the Opinions of these excellent Commentators, yet, on the Whole, I am to acknowledge myself greatly obliged to them, and that even more and oftener than I have had Opportunity to name it.

Beside these, I have been at the Pains of examining many other of the Critics, and have adopted several of their Opinions. Many others, whom I have not been able to see, and many of the Quotations I have taken on Credit from *Salmasius*, who has carefully collected them, and whose Fidelity I have never once found Occasion to question: His Opinions, indeed, I have in some Places been obliged to dissent from, as I have every where ventured to think for myself, and determine myself by the Bodies themselves which are described, whenever I could be so happy to have them before me. And, indeed, any one who will study Nature's self, will often see wherein he must dissent, not only from the best Critics, but even from the best Authors in Natural History.

By these Means, and with these Assistances, it is, that I have undertaken to give a new Edition of the *Greek* Text, in which whatever may be the Service I have done, I promise myself I shall, at least, be liable to no Censure; since tho' I have filled up all the Defects, and amended the Errors, so as to make the Work now plain, intelligible, and easy to be read, I have every where in the Notes mentioned where the Lacunæ were, and what were the Words that I have ventured to alter, so that this Edition yet leaves the Text for those who would attempt new Emendations, in the same Condition with the others, as by referring to the Notes, it will always be seen how I found it. To this let me add, that in order to leave the Author as much himself as possible, I have been most scrupulously sparing in the Alterations, which I could else have wish'd much more numerous. This the learned Reader will see in some few Places, where, though I have left the Original standing, as I found it, I have yet, by the Translation, shewn how I thought a few Letters might have been altered to Advantage. I am sorry to add, that, notwithstanding all the Corrections of the Press, there are yet, here and there, some Errors of a Letter or so in the Text, I think, however, there are fewer of them than in most other Works lately printed in this Language, and as they are but trifling, the *Greek* Reader will easily see what they are, and others they will not concern.

Thus much for the *Greek* Text. In regard to the *English*, I have only to observe, that as my Intent was to render the Work as intelligible to the *English* as to the learned Reader, I have not tied myself down to a bare verbal Translation. This Author is remarkably concise in his Expression, and want of Words has in many Places helped to render him less easily intelligible. I have, therefore, to make his Sense the more evident, attempted to give, not barely his Words, but his Meaning, and in many

Places have translated a single Syllable into a whole Sentence, by giving, where that Syllable referred to something said before, a short Recapitulation of the Matter referred to, and by that means preserving the necessary Connection of Thought, without which, what followed might have appeared obscure.

Besides this, in order to serve the great End of making the Work as easy and intelligible as possible, I have divided the Whole into a Number of Sections, which are no other than so many distinct separate Sentences, often having not the least Reference to, or Connection with one another, and this is done, not only in the *English*, but in the *Greek* also, by which the Translation may be every where readily compared with the Original, and the Reader prevented from being confounded, by imagining the Author is carrying on his Reasonings on any particular Subject, when perhaps he has suddenly dropt it, and is gone on to a different one. I promise myself it will appear, that I have followed the Author's Meaning closely and regularly in this Particular; and yet in many Places, where the Sentences are here made to terminate, there is not in the other Editions so much as a Stop: How much this must, in a continued Treatise, before rendered too obscure by many other Defects, at first sight, confound even a judicious Reader, is easy to imagine.

I have chosen to give the Translation in *English* rather than *Latin*, partly because there are already many *Latin* Translations of this Work, and all very much and very deservedly censured, the Translators many of them having, in numerous Instances, only given a Word, that in the *Latin* expressed some one Sense of that they were translating from the *Greek*, and never given themselves the Trouble of so much as attempting to give the Author's Meaning, and partly, because one great Intent of this Edition was, to make the Treatise as universally read and understood here as possible: And it may be observed, that those who are able to read *Latin* Translations to Advantage, generally are able to have made them, and therefore are above having Recourse to them. In the Notes, however, has been the principal Labour; in these, beside giving an Account of the Lacunæ that are filled up, and Alterations that are made, I have endeavoured, partly by Examinations of the Bodies themselves, which are described, partly by Comparison of the Words with those of others of the Antients, and partly by the Assistance of the Critics, to elucidate, explain, and account for, whatever the Author has left us. How far I have been so happy to succeed in this, is left to the Determination of the learned Reader; what I have offered are given but as Conjectures, and, at this distance of Time, it is impossible that this ever should be perfectly done.

To the Authors general Systems I have added those of the later Naturalists; and in this, it is surprising to see how much those of the best of them agree with his; and to every Gem, Stone, Earth, or other Substance he describes, I have added the more modern History of it. And in this we shall also be surprised to see how much was so early known. Beside these, I have occasionally taken in many other fossile Bodies which he has not described, in order to render the Whole as useful as a Treatise in so small a Compass might be. In these Things it may be necessary to observe, that I have no where servilely tied myself down to the Opinions of any particular Author: In the Systems I have in general followed the late excellent Dr. *Woodward*, a Man ever to be remembered with the highest Veneration by all who make these Things their Study, and who has, perhaps given us more real Knowledge in the Fossile World than all who went before him;

As the Dwarf, however, on the Giant's Shoulders, there are some Things, perhaps, in which a much less Genius may, by the Help of the Fund of Knowledge he has left, see yet something farther, and in such, and such only, I have ventured to dissent from him. In the Accounts of particular Substances, I have not omitted what was to be collected from Authors most to be depended on, but have made the Bodies themselves my great Instructors; and every where, where I could have them before me, formed my Descriptions from them.

Whatever may be the Reception of this Attempt in the learned World, this I can with great Justice affirm, that be the Defects of it what they will, Labour has not been wanting in it. If my Intentions are so far answered, that the Judicious look on it as a Thing of any real Use in the Study of Fossils, or if it spirit up any body else to give us Editions of the Works of the Antients on other Subjects in the same manner, as I find my own particular Avocations will not permit me to engage in more, at the utmost, than those on this, I shall account myself very happy, that I have ventured to break the Ice, and point out a Way to make the Works of these early Naturalists generally useful.

Θ E O-

ΘΕΟΦΡΑΣΤΟΥ
ΤΟΥ ΕΡΕΣΙΟΥ
ΠΕΡΙ ΤΩΝ
ΛΙΘΩΝ
ΒΙΒΛΙΟΝ.

THEOPHRASTUS's
HISTORY
OF
STONES.

ΘΕΟΦΡΑΣΤΟΥ
ΤΟΥ ΕΡΕΣΙΟΥ
ΠΕΡΙ ΤΩΝ
᾿ΛΙΘΩΝ[a]
ΒΙΒΛΙΟΝ.

α'. ΤΩΝ ἐν τῇ γῇ συνιϛαμένων, τὰ μέν ἐςιν ὕδατ۞· τὰ δὲ γῆς.

β'. [b]Ὕδατ۞ μὲ τὰ μεταλλευόμενα, καθάπερ ἄργυρος, ὺ χρυσ۞, ὺ τἄλλα γῆς δὲ, λίθ۞ τε ὺ

---

[a] THIS excellent Author, notwithstanding that he has made the Title of the Treatise before us promise no more than an Account of *Stones*, we shall find hereafter, did not mean to confine himself in it strictly and literally to discourse of only that Part of the fossile Kingdom generally understood by this Name, but to take into his Consideration, at the same Time, all those other mineral Substances which appeared to him to be formed of Matter of a like Kind with them; as the various *Earths*, &c. in short all the native Fossils, which, according to his Philosophy, had *Earth*, not *Water*, for the Basis of their Formation.

[b] Our Author's general System of the fossile World I shall not, in these Times of greater Knowledge, attempt to vindicate in all its Parts, but must do him the Justice to observe, that it was far from being either absurd, or improbable, at the Time when he wrote, when the Sciences, to which the present Age owes its Improvements in Natural Knowledge, were so little understood, and so few of the Experiments, which have now given Light into

THEOPHRASTUS's HISTORY OF STONES.

I. OF Things formed in the Earth, some have their Origin from *Water*, others from *Earth*

II. [b] *Water* is the Basis of Metals, as Silver, Gold, and the rest, *Earth* of Stones, as well the more

---

it, had been made, and that it carries, at least, an equal Air of Probability, with many that have been since formed, and is absolutely more succinctly, clearly, and philosophically delivered than any of them all.

The Principles of mixed Bodies, as well those of the *fossile*, as of the *vegetable* and *animal* Kingdoms, are indeed so intimately mixed, and closely combined together, at their original Formation, that we are not to wonder, an Author, who wrote in such early Times, was not clearly acquainted with the exact Manner of their Composition. Those who have followed him, even after the Discoveries of many succeeding Ages, and with the Assistance of Chemistry, the best and surest of all Means of judging, and which, whatever some Men of fertile Imaginations may have thought, we have no sound Reason to believe was much known in his Time, have yet been of late found to have run into great Errors about them, and even those of the present and last Age, who have been able to discover their Mistakes, and have the Advantage of yet greater and farther Improvements in that Science, if they will speak

(4)

ἴσα λίθων πεπτότερα. ἢ εἴ τινες δὴ τῆς γῆς αὐτῆς ἰδιώτεραι φύσεις εἰσὶν, ἢ χρώμασιν, ἢ λειότησιν, ἢ πυκνότησιν, ἢ ἐξ ἄλλῃ τινὶ δυνάμει.

---

frankly and ingenuously, must own, that though they have discovered the Errors of their Predecessors, and are certain they are nearer the real Knowledge of the Mysteries of Nature than those of any other Age have been, they yet are sensible, that they are only making farther and farther Advances toward what, perhaps, it is not in human Nature ever perfectly to know.

Chemical Analyses, when judiciously and carefully made, are unquestionably the surest and best Methods we can use, towards the Attainment of that Knowledge; and yet, how imperfect our best Discoveries by these may appear to the industrious and ingenious of future Ages, may be guessed by the Errors we can discover in those of but a few before us.

When Chemistry became, some Time ago, better understood and more practised than it had probably ever before been, the Professors of it, finding a certain Number of different Substances, into which almost all mixed Bodies were resolvible, immediately looked upon these as fixed and unalterable in themselves, and as they found them, in a Manner, in all mixed Bodies, they determined that they were the true *Principles* or *Elements* of which all Bodies were compounded, and fixed their Number, and their Names, *viz.* That they were five, *Spirit, Sulphur, Salt, Water,* and *Earth.* Here then the whole Work seemed effected, the Secrets of Nature opened, and the true, fixed, and unalterable *Principles* of mixed Bodies clearly known.

But what Figure does this boasted Philosophy, this Set of Principles now make? when our own Experience, and the Discoveries of later Chemists give us even the unquestionable Testimony of our Senses, that no less than three of the five are so far from deserving the Name of *Principles* or *Elements*, that they are themselves mixed Bodies, and resolvible with proper Care into other distinct and different Substances. For the fine Chemistry, which has

precious, as the common; and of the various *Earths* of peculiar Kinds, whether remarkable for Colour, Smoothness, Density, or whatever other Quality.

---

brought *Sulphur* out of a mixed Body, will also separate that *Sulphur* into *Salt, Water,* and *Earth*; and when it has extracted from another, that *Salt,* they esteemed so true a *Principle,* will afterwards reduce it also into *Water* and *Earth,* and *Spirit,* we now find, is no other than Oil attenuated by Salts, and dissolved in Water. This appears by this plain and easy Experiment of Mr *Boyle's, viz.* If Spirit of Wine be mixed with ten or twelve times it's Weight of Water, and set in a cool Place, the Salts will fly off, the Water mix itself with the Water in the Mixture, and the Oil be left swimming at the Top.

Instead of the five Principles, therefore, of the Chemists before us, farther Discoveries have reduced us to a Necessity of owning only two, visible, obvious, and the Objects of our Senses, and even these two may perhaps hereafter be proved to be more nearly allied to each other than we at present imagine; these are *Water* and *Earth,* the very *Principles,* and the *only ones,* acknowledged by this excellent Author, whose Works I am offering my Remarks on, and who, to his immortal Honour be it recorded, discovered that by Reason and Philosophy alone, which we owe the Knowledge of to a thousand tedious Experiments.

His System, though founded on this excellent Basis, I do not, as I before observed, attempt to justify; Observations, which it was impossible for him to have made, have given us the Testimony of our Senses, that Metals do contain more or less of an absolute, genuine, and vitrifiable Earth, and Stones, it is as certain, are never wholly divested of that Water which once served to bring their constituent Parts together.

But to return to the Principles of mixed Bodies. Reason informs us, that these two, *Water* and *Earth,* alone can never have made all the Differences, and Virtues of them; we are compelled therefore to acknowledge a third, as obvious to our Reason as the others to our Senses, an active Something, to give that to the Mass, which Water and Earth alone could not. This unknown Principle is what

γ΄. Περὶ μὲν ὖν τ̅ μεταλλοειδῶν ἐν ἄλλοις τεθεώ-
ρη]. περὶ δὲ τύτων, νῦν λέγωμεν.

δ΄. Ἅπαντα ὖν ταῦτα χρὴ νομίζειν, ὡς ἁπλῶς
εἰπεῖν, ἐκ καθαρᾶς τινὸς ξυνεςάναι καὶ ὁμαλῆς ὕλης,
εἴτε ῥοῆς, εἴτε διηθήσεως διά τινὸς γινομένης, εἴτε, ὡς
ἀνωτέρω εἴρη], καὶ κατ᾿ ἄλλον τρόπον ἐκκεκριμένης·
τάχα γὰρ ἐνδεχε], τὰ μὲν ὕτως, τὰ δ᾽ ἐκείνως, τὰ
δ᾽ ἄλλως[c].

---

some Chemists have called *Acid*, and the Metaphysicians *Fire*, Words which in their general and common Acceptation convey Ideas very different from those we mean to express by them on this Occasion, but which we must be indulged in the Use of, till a more perfect Knowledge of the Thing we mean to express has taught us to give it a more determinate Name

[c] The Author has here justly, clearly, and succinctly given the general Manner, in which the constituent Matter of Earths and Stones has been brought together, and hinted at the various other Means by which it is done in other particular Cases.

The two general Ways he allows are by *Afflux* and *Percolation*, and nothing is more certain than that, by these two Methods, the two great Classes of the Bodies he is here to treat of, have been brought into a State of Formation; the *Earths* and *Stones* of Strata by *Afflux* and the *Crystals*, *Spars*, and other Bodies of that Kind, by *Percolation*.

The Agent, in the first of these Cases, has been Gravity, and in the other, the continual passing of Water through the solid Strata

When we look up to the original Formation of these Substances, we find the Particles, of which they were to be composed, in loose Atoms, diffused, and floating in that confused and irregular Mass of Matter (for that is evidently

III. The *Metals* have been confidered in another Work, the *Stones* and *Earths* of various Kinds, therefore, are to be the Subject of this Treatife.

IV. All thefe we are (plainly fpeaking) to judge formed by the Concretion of Matter pure and equal in its conftituent Parts, which has been brought together in that State by mere *Afflux*, or by means of fome Kind of *Percolation*; or feparated, as before obferved, from the impurer Matter it was once among, in fome other Manner; for perhaps it is effected in fome Cafes by one, and in others by other of thefe Means

---

the Senfe of the Word תהום which we find tranflated the *Deep*) out of which this Earth was to be formed. The great Agent in gathering thefe fcattered Atoms into a Mafs, and feparating them from the Water they were before floating in, feems to have been what in the *Mofaic* Account of the Creation is called the *Spirit of the Creator*.

On the Action of this powerful Minifter, the conftituent Particles of Matter were collected into a Body, by their own Weight feparated themfelves from the Fluid they before fwam in, and fubfided, fome fooner, fome later, in Proportion to their different Gravities. By this Means the Particles of Stone, for Inftance, precipitated themfelves and formed a Stratum entire, homogene, and pure, before thofe of Clay began to fubfide, which afterwards falling in a Mafs on the Stratum of Stone already formed, conftituted another of Clay over it, and after all this, a Quantity of yet lighter Matter, fettling on the Surface of this laft formed Stratum, added to that another of what we call vegetable Mould, or fomething of that Kind. In this Manner were the different Strata of the Earth formed, and the Difference of the Matter, which was to fubfide in different Parts of the Globe, made that almoft infinite Variety to be found in the Matter of the Strata.

This original Structure of the Earth, however, we are not now to expect to find it in, the univerfal Deluge has made many and wonderful Alterations in it, which are now

(8)

έ. Ἀφ' ὧν δὴ καὶ τὸ λεῖον, ἢ τὸ πυκνὸν, ἢ τὸ ςιλπνὸν, καὶ διαφανές, καὶ τᾶλλα τὰ τοιαῦτα ἔχουσι. ἢ ὅσον ἂν ἢ ὁμαλέςερον, ἓ καθαρώτερον ἔλαςον ἢ, τοσύτω ἢ ταῦτα μᾶλλον ὑπάρχει.

---

every where obvious to our Senses, and are everlasting Records of that fatal Catastrophe, of which the Earth, in the Condition we now see it, is but the Ruins.

There are many and incontestible Proofs, that the Surface of the Globe, to a Depth beyond what we ever dig, was, in the Time of that fatal Calamity, dissolved and reduced nearly into the Condition it was in at the Time of its original Formation; the stony, mineral, and even metalline, as well as earthy Matter, floating in the Waters that then covered it, in separate Particles, these, when the Tumult of that Immensity of Waters began to cease, were by the same Laws of Gravity again precipitated, and subsided in Proportion to their different Weights; but this not in their original Purity, for the metalline and other heterogene Matter, nay and even extraneous Substances, the Shells of Sea Fishes, &c. if of about equal Gravity, subsided among the stony Matter they were before suspended amidst, and made a Part of the Stratum that Precipitation formed; the lighter Matters, the Earths, Clays, &c. afterwards subsided into other Strata over these, and with them other extraneous Particles and Substances of Gravities like theirs. And thus the present Surface of the Globe was formed, in Strata of different Kinds, and that again according to their different Gravities; except where the Motion of the Waters prevented this Regularity, by lodging sometimes on lighter Strata already formed, other whole Beds of weightier Matter, which its immense and irresistible Force had taken up, and now in its abating suffered to subside again. This then, with the Alterations made by Earthquakes afterwards bursting, and elevating or sinking the Strata in many Places, is the present Condition of the outer Crust of this Earth to a certain Depth, far within which perhaps all our Researches lie, and in the Mass of

V. From the Differences of the constituent Matter, and Manner of its Coalescence, the *Concrete* assumes its different *Qualities*, as *Smoothness, Density, Brightness, Transparency,* and the like, and according as it is more pure and equal, the more does it partake of them.

---

which we find, according to the System of our Author, the Strata of Stone and Earth, formed by the Concretion of Matter, equal in Weight and many other of its Properties, and brought together in that State by mere Afflux, by means of the Action of Gravity, and in the perpendicular Fissures of those Strata, and some other Places, Crystals, Spars, and other like Substances, separated by Percolation from the arenaceous, argillaceous, and other Matter, among which they subsided in their separated Particles; and brought together there by the continual draining of Water through the solid Strata, which in its Passage had taken them up with it, and there deserted them in different Manners, and left them to assume the Figures which are the natural and necessary Consequences of their Concretions

These then are the two general Methods of Formation of these Bodies mentioned by our Author; the various others, which he hints at as taking Place in some particular Cases, are too numerous to be all recited here. Terrestrial and sparry Matter, washed from the Strata by the Water of Springs in their Passage, and subsiding at some Distance from their Source, round various Substances in Form of Incrustations, is one. Matter of a like Kind, and separated in a like Manner, dropping from the Tops of Caverns with the Water, and either deserted by it at the Top, and left in Form of Icycles or *Stalactæ*, or at the Bottom, and left in Masses called *Stalagmitæ*, or *Dropstones*, is another very frequent one. Many others there also are, but the Bodies formed by these, as well as those, though not brought together by mere Percolation, or mere Afflux, are however, in general, of the Number of the Bodies formed of Particles originally brought together by the one or the other of these Means, and therefore very justly redu-

ς'. Τὸ γὰ ὅλον, ὡς ἂν ἀκριβείας ἔχῃ κ̄τ' τ̄ ζύςα-
σιν ἡ πῆξις, ὕτως ἀκολυθεῖ κ̀ τὰ ἀπ' ἐκείνων.

ζ'. [d] Ἡ γ̀ πῆξις, τοῖς μὲν ἀπὸ θερμῦ, τοῖς δ' ἀπὸ
ψυχρῦ γίνε]. κωλύᾳ γ̀ ἴσως ὐδὲν ἔνια γένη λίθων ὑφ'
ἑκατέρων ζυνίςαςθ τύτων. ἐπεὶ τάτε τ̃ γῆς ἅπαν[α
δόξᾳεν ὑπὸ πυρὸς, ἐπείπερ ἐν τοῖς ἐναντίοις ἡ πῆξις
κ̀ ἡ τῆξις.

―――――――――

cible under them as general Heads What the Author adds of the various Stones and Earths, thus formed, owing their various Qualities to the Variety and Purity of the conſtituent Matter, and of the Manner of Concretion, is plain, evident, and inconteſtible.

[d] The Author has here, in his accuſtomed clear and ſuccinct Manner, given his Opinion in regard to the Cauſes of the Concretion of that Matter he had before deſcribed the Nature of, for the Formation of the Bodies which are to be the Subject of the preſent Treatiſe

The certain and immediate Cauſe of the Coheſion of theſe Particles, which had before, by their Gravity, been precipitated from among the fluid Matter they were at firſt ſuſpended in, was that univerſal Property in Matter called Attraction The Preſſure of the circumambient Atmoſphere may ſerve to account for the Coheſion of large Maſſes of Matter, but the minute Contacts of leſſer Particles of it, which ſometimes cohere with a Force almoſt infinitely greater than the Preſſure upon them can be ſuppoſed to influence, reduce us to a Neceſſity of having Recourſe to this other Power of Attraction, a Property in all Matter, by which the Particles of Bodies draw one another with a certain Force, which acts infinitely more

VI. On the whole, the more perfectly the *Concretion* was formed, and the more *equal* in its constituent Parts the concreting Matter was, the more does the *Concrete* possess the peculiar Properties which are owing to that Equality

VII [d] The Concretion is, in some of these Substances, owing to *Heat*, and in others to *Cold*. There is perhaps nothing to hinder but that the Coalescence of some Kinds of *Stones* may be occasioned by the one, and of others by the other of these Causes: though that of the *Earths* of all Kinds seems owing only to *Heat*. From these contrary Causes, however, may happen the Concretion or Dissipation of contrary Substances.

---

intensely at the Contact, or extremely near it, than at any determinate Distance

How far the Heat, which is apparently manifest to our Senses at great Depths in the Earth, and is from thence, and from much greater Depths than we are ever likely to have Opportunities of being acquainted with, continually passing upwards to the Surface, may have been concerned in dissipating the remaining Part of the Water, which had served to bring the Particles of Stones and Earths together, and, by that means, been instrumental to the bringing them into their present State, and how far the Cold about the Surface may have assisted in the Formation of others, by preventing the Dissipation or farther Rise of their constituent Particles, which had been washed from among the Matter of the Strata by the Water which continually also ascends from below towards the Surface, incessantly pervading them, and detaching and bearing up with it these Particles from among them, is a Subject of too nice Enquiry, and too long to be particularly decided here. The bare Mention of it may however serve to explain in what Manner Heat and Cold may be concerned in the reducing some of the fossile Substances into the State we find them in, and how Heat would have destroyed the

(12)

η'. Ἰδιότητες δὲ πλείους εἰσὶν ἐν τοῖς λίθοις· ἐν γὰρ τῇ γῇ χρώμασί τε, καὶ γλιχρότητι, καὶ λειότητι, καὶ πυκνότητι, καὶ τοῖς τοιούτοις αἱ ῥοαὶ διάφοροι κἂν δὲ τὰ ἄλλα σπάνια[c].

θ'. Τοῖς δὲ λίθοις αὗταί τε καὶ πρὸς ταύταις[f] αἱ κατὰ τὰς δυνάμεις, τῦ τε ποιεῖν, ἢ πάσχειν, ἢ τῦ μὴ πάσχειν· τηκτοὶ γὰρ, οἱ δ' ἄτηκτοι καὶ καυστοὶ, οἱ δ' ἄκαυστοι.

very Means of Coalescence in those Subjects, to the Formation of which Cold has, according to this Philosophy, been essential; and Cold, on the contrary, must have prevented what Heat uninterrupted might have had Power of doing in the others

[c] The Author, having now treated of the constituent Matter of these fossile Substances, and the Manner and Causes of its Coalescence, in order to their Formation, comes here to the Consideration of the Differences of the distinct Classes and separate Species of them And these he very justly and philosophically deduces from the different Matter of which they are formed, and the various Elaborations it has passed in the Affluxes by which it has been brought together. The terrestrial Matter, which serves as the Basis of their Formation, he observes, is very commonly found differing in Colour, Density, &c. and hence the Stones formed of it have very frequently these Differences, which make the many various Species of the

VIII. There are in *Stones* of different Kinds many peculiar Qualities, which arise from this, that there are many very great Differences both in the Matter and Manner of the Affluxes of the terrestrial Particles from which they were formed; of which those in regard to Colour, Tenacity, Smoothness, Density, and the like Accidents, are frequent, though those in other more remarkable Properties, are not so common [e].

IX. These Qualities *Stones* have, therefore, from the common Differences of the Matter and Manner of the Affluxes of their constituent Parts: But besides these, they have others [f] which arise from the more peculiar Powers of their concreted Masses; such are their acting upon other Bodies, or being subject, or not subject to be acted upon by them. Thus some are fusible, others will never liquify in the Fire; some may be calcined, others are incombustible;

---

common Strata of them, but that there are also other Varieties in this coalescent Matter, in regard to more peculiar Qualities, which are more rarely found, but which, wherever they are, make Differences in the Body formed from them, of other and more remarkable Kinds, as he goes on to shew in their proper Places.

Some Editions of this Author have it ποιαὶ διαφοραὶ and others πολλαὶ διαφοραὶ in the last Line of this Sentence; the ποιαὶ διαφοραὶ is a very rational and judicious Alteration of *De Laet*'s, and in all Probability was the true original Reading.

[f] The common Differences of the more frequent and large Masses of Stone having been now accounted for, from the frequent Diversities of the Earths from which they were formed, which are found to differ, like them, in the common Accidents of Colour, &c. and even much more than they, in every Pit, the Author now proceeds to enumerate the Differences of a more remarkable Kind, observable in the more rare and valuable Species, and oc-

(14)

κ̀ ἄλλα τύποις ὅμοια. κ̀ ἐν αὐτῇ τῇ καύσει κ̀
πυρώσει πλείους ἔχοντες διαφοράς.

i. ἔνιοι ὴ τοῖς χρώμασιν ἐξομοιοῦν λέγουσι δυνά-
μενοι τὸ ὕδωρ, ὥσπερ ἡ σμάραγδ^Θ. οἱ δ' ὅλως ἀπο-
λιθοῦν τὰ τιθέμενα εἰς ἑαυτοὺς ἕτεροι ὴ ὀλίγω τινα

---

cafioned, according to his Syftem, by Diverfities of lefs frequent, and therefore more remarkable Qualities in the Matter from which they were formed, which, together with the more fingular Operations of Nature, in feparating and afterwards bringing that Matter into a Mafs, have imparted to the formed Subftance *Qualities*, or, as he chufes to exprefs it by a Word of greater Signification, *Powers* more fingular and obfervable than thofe occafioned by lefs effential and more common Varieties in both.

ε After affigning the Caufes of the various Figures and Qualities as well of the common, as the more rare and precious Kinds of *Stones* and *Earths*, the Author here enters into a Detail of what they are.

The Emerald is the Stone whofe Properties he begins with; but as he only hints, in this Place, at what he more particularly explains himfelf upon fome Pages after, I fhall referve what I have to offer, on this Subject, to that Part of the Work, where there will be a more immediate Opportunity of comparing it with his own Words

The Stone he next mentions, and of which he has recorded the petrifying Power, but not the Name, is the *Lapis Affius*, or *Sarcophagus* The *Affian*, or Flefh-confuming Stone The *Sarcophagus, Boet* 403 *Afius vel Affius Lapis, Chailt.* 251. *Sarcophagus, five Affius Lapis, De Laet* 133 *Affius Lapis, Salmaf in Solin* 847 *Plin* Book 36 Chap 17

This was a Stone much known, and ufed among the *Greeks* in their Sepultures, and by them cal'ed σαρκοφαγος from its Power of confuming the Flefh of Bodies buried in it, which it is faid to have perfectly effected in forty Days and in others, other such particular Properties are observable: To which it may be added, that in the Action of the Fire on them, they also shew many Differences

X. Some are said to have a Power of making Water become of their own Colour, as the *Emerald*. Others of petrifying, or converting wholly into Stone, whatever is put into Vessels made of them. Others have

---

This Property it was much famed for, and all the ancient Naturalists mention it, but the other, of turning into Stone Things put into Vessels of it, has been recorded only by this Author and *Mucianus*, from whom *Pliny* has copied it, and from him some few only of the later Naturalists. The Account *Mutianus* gives of it is, that it converted into Stone the Shoes of Persons buried in it, as also the Utensils, which it was in some Places customary to bury with the Body, particularly those the Persons while living had most delighted in. The Utensils he mentions are such as must have been made of many different Materials, whence it appears, that this Stone had a Power of consuming only Flesh, but that its petrifying Quality extended to Substances of very different Kinds. Whether it really possessed this last Quality, or not, has been much doubted, and many have been afraid, from its supposed Improbability, to record it. What has much encouraged a Disbelief of it is *Mutianus*'s Account of its thus taking Place on Subjects of different Kinds and Textures. But this, in my Opinion, is no Objection at all, and the whole Account, very probably, true. Petrifactions, in those early Days, might not be distinguished from Incrustations of sparry or stony Matter, as even, with many People, they are not to this Day; the Incrustations of Spar on Moss and other Substances, in some Springs, being yet called by many petrified Moss, &c. and these might easily be formed on Substances enclosed in Vessels, made of this Stone, by Water, if its Situation was in the Way of its passing through its Pores, dislodging from the common Matter of the Stone, and carrying with it sparry or other such Particles, and afterwards

(16)

ποιεῖν. οἱ δὲ βασανίζειν τ' ἄργυρον, ὥσπερ ἥτε καλυμένη λίθος Ἡράκλεια, καὶ ἡ Λυδή.

ιά. Θαυμασιωτάτη δὲ καὶ μεγίστη δύναμις, εἴπερ ἀληθές, ἡ τ' τίκτων [h].

---

leaving them, in Form of Incrustations, on whatever it found in its Way, and by this Means Things made of Substances of ever so different Natures and Textures, which happened to be enclosed, and in the Way of the Passage of the Water, would be equally incrusted with, and in Appearance turned to Stone, without Regard to their different Configuration of Pores or Parts.

The Place where this Stone was dug was near *Assos*, a City in *Lycia*, from whence it had its Name; and *Boetius* informs us, that in that Country, and in some Parts of the East, there were also Stones of this Kind, which, if tied to the Bodies of living Persons, would, in the same Manner, consume their Flesh.

The Stones mentioned next, as having an attractive Power, are the Load-stone, Amber, &c. but as both these and the Lapis Lydius are hereafter described more at large by the Author, I shall reserve to that Place what I have to add in regard to them.

[h] This is one of the many Passages for which this excellent Author has been censured by Persons who had never sufficiently studied, or, perhaps even read him (as I hope to prove has been the general Case in the Accusations he has been subject to) and which has been as much misunderstood and misrepresented as perhaps any one of them all.

Pliny has given the Handle to the Accusations of him in this Place, by saying, that he and *Mutianus* believed there were Stones which brought forth young. *Idem Theophrastus et Mutianus esse aliquos lapides qui pariant credunt.* This has been a sufficient Source of Censures on this Author, most of those who quote, or mention him, never having given themselves the Trouble of learning any thing more of him than what *Pliny* has told them; as this, and many other Passages, frequently quoted from him, to be

hereafter

an attractive Quality. And others serve for the Trial of Metals, as that called the *Heraclian*, or *Lydian* Stone.

XI. The greatest, however, and most wonderful of all the Qualities of *Stones* is that (if the Accounts of it are true) of those which bring forth young.

---

hereafter considered, will abundantly prove. But, with *Pirn*'s Leave, I must observe, that I find no Reason here to imagine, that *Theophrastus* ever believed any such Thing; he mentions it, on the contrary, as a Thing which he did not believe, but which, though, as it was generally reputed true, and a very remarkable *Property* of a Stone, he could not avoid mentioning in a Place where he was professedly writing on that Subject, but would not however let pass, even though he did allow it a Place, without frankly expressing his own Suspicion that it was but an idle and groundless Story.

The Stone meant is the Ætites, or Eagle Stone, the *Ætites, seu Aquilinus Lapis, Worm.* 77 *Charlt.* 31. *Lapis Ætites, Boet.* 375. *De Laet* 114. *Ætitæ, Gesn de Lap.* 10. famous for its imaginary Virtues in assisting in Delivery, preventing Abortions, and, which it at least equally possesses, discovering Thieves. That the general Opinion was long what our Author records as reported of it, is easily proved, and we cannot wonder at that's being firmly believed, when we find such Virtues as the other of choaking Thieves, &c. as certainly credited, and recorded by the gravest Authors.

That it was, long after, as well as before this Author's Time, believed to have this Property of bringing forth, is evident from the Words *prægnans, gravidus Uterus,* ἐγκύμων, &c. so constantly used in describing it. *Pliny* says of it, *est autem lapis iste prægnans intus, quum quatias, alio velut in utero sonante.* *Dioscorides,* ἀετίτης λίθος ὡς ἕτερῳ ἐγκύμων λίθῳ ὑπάρχων. And almost numberless Instances might be brought of the earliest as well as later Authors using the like Expressions, and evidently testifying, that the Stone was, or had been generally believed to possess this so remarkable Quality, and which perhaps this Author, who is accused of believing, was the very first who ever doubted.

ιϛ'. Γνωριμώτερα ϳ τ̃, κϳ ἐν πλείοσι κϳ τὰς ἐργασίας. γλυπτοὶ ϳὰ ἔνιοι, κϳ τορνωτοὶ, κϳ περιτοί. τῶν ϳ ὐδὲ ὅλως ἄπτετ) σιδήριον, ἐνίων ϳ κακῶς κϳ μόλις.[1]

In order to the establishing a more rational Account of the Formation of this Stone, it may not be amiss here to look into the Formation of Pebbles and Flints in general, of which Class of Stones this is a Species, and by which we shall find, that the Callimus, or included Stone, is instead of a young one, indeed the older of the two, and has had some Share in the Formation of its Parent, as the outer one was generally esteemed, though that has nothing to do with the Production of it

The Flints and Pebbles, we now every where see, were all formed in the Waters of the Deluge, by the mere Afflux of their constituent Matter, the first Concretion of this was generally in small Quantity, and formed a little Lump or Nodule, this afterwards encreased in Bigness by the Application of fresh Matter, in different Quantities, and at different Times to it If this new Matter happened to be of different Textures and Appearances, the separate Quantities, that at times affixed themselves, became different Crusts of various Colours, as may be observed frequently in our common Pebbles; if of the same Nature and Colour, and affixed nearly all at once, the Apposition became, imperceptible afterwards, and the Mass formed of the whole appeared a Flint, or Pebble, of regular and similar Substance and if, lastly, this Matter, before its Application, had received other various coloured Affluxes into it, it shews them in the Concrete, in irregular Lines and Striæ, and becomes an Agate, Onyx, or other such Stone. In all these Cases the Matter first formed into a Mass, yet remains in Form of a central Nucleus, in or near the Middle, of the Stone, according to the equal or irregular Quanti-

XII. But the moſt known and general Properties of Stones are their ſeveral Fitneſſes for the various Kinds of Work. Some of them are proper for engraving on, others may be ſhaped by the Turner's Tools, others may be cut or ſawed. Some alſo there are which no Iron Inſtruments will touch; and others which are very difficultly, or ſcarce at all to be cut by them [1].

---

ty of the additional Matter which formed each Cruſt, this being ſometimes all of the ſame Colour with that Nucleus, made it unperceivable, but ſometimes, as before obſerved, was of different Colours, and left it evident to the Eye.

This Nucleus in ſome, indeed moſt of theſe Maſſes being of the Texture of the reſt, has remained in its Place, and become a viſible Spot of equal Hardneſs and Beauty with the reſt of the Stone, in others, after the Application of ſome, or all the outer Cruſts, it has ſhrunk into a ſmaller Compaſs, detached itſelf from the inner Cruſt, and become a looſe, ſeparate Stone, rolling about in the Cavity, now too large for it, and rattling in it when ſhaken. And this is our Ætites, and the central Nucleus ſo detached, and ſhrunk, its Callimus. In others, this central Nucleus has fallen into looſe, ſandy, or earthy Matter, and remaining in that Form, looſe in its Cavity, made what is called the Geodes, or baſtard Eagle Stone. The Geodes, and the Eagle Stone, ſo much renowned for Virtues, and ſo fabulouſly talked of as to its Origin, are therefore no other than common Pebbles, the central Nuclei of which have, from the different Nature and Texture of the Matter they were formed of, detached themſelves from the ſuperadded Cruſts, and either ſhrunk, on becoming more dry, into ſmaller Dimenſions, or fallen into the original Grit, or ſandy Matter, of which they were firſt compoſed.

[1] I cannot but obſerve from this Paſſage of our Author, that, ſo early as in his Time, not only very many Species of precious Stones were in Uſe, and their different Degrees of Hardneſs familiarly known, but that the various Manners of working them were alſo well underſtood, even better

(20)

ιγ. Εἰσὶ ἢ πλείες κ̓ ἄλλαι κ̓ ταύτας ἰδιότητας διαφοραί. αἱ μ̃ ἓν κ̓ χρώματα, κ̓ τὰς σκληρότητας, κ̓ μαλακότητας κ̓ λειότητας, κ̓ τἄλλα τὰ τοιαῦτα, διὰ τὸ πεῖτον, πλείοσιν ὑπάρχουσιν [k]

ιέ. Καὶ ἐνίοις γε κ̓ τόπον ὅλον, ἐξ ὧν δὴ κ̓ διωνομασμέναι λιθοτομίαι, Παρίων τε κ̓ Πεντελικῶν, κ̓ Χίων τε κ̓ Θηβαικῶν.

---

than in the succeeding Ages, for he is here clear in the Distinction between the γλυ-ʃω and τορ υἰοἱ which much later Writers of his Nation are very justly accused of having confounded, for the γλυ-ʃω and τορνευτὸ of the Greeks, however confusedly misunderstood by some of them, and used as synonymous Terms by others, are really Words of distinct and determinate Sense, and signify the *Cælatura* and *Tornatura* of the *Latins*, which, I think, it is evident from this Passage, was well known to this Author, however it came to be forgotten afterwards.

[k] The Author, having now mentioned several very remarkable Properties in Stones, and their general Characters as to Difference of Texture, from the different Ways they are to be worked on, proceeds here to relate the many other Differences they have in their several peculiar Qualities, which they owe, as he has before established it, to the different Matter and Manner of the Affluxes of their constituent Parts, and such of which as arise from the more common Varieties of terrestrial Matter, in Colour, &c. he again observes, are common to many and great Quantities.

This is only repeating, in its due Place, and at the Head of that Class of Stones to which it properly belongs, what he had before given as a Part of his general System. it was long, however, before this Passage was in a Condition to be thus understood, for after the Word ταυτας, there was by Defect in the Copy a Gap left, which some Editors had filled up with the Word διαφοραὶ only, but others, finding

XIII. There are also, besides these, many other Differences observable in them, according to their several Qualities, of which those in regard to Colour, Hardness, Softness, Smoothness, and the like Accidents, because of the Number and Diversity of those Qualities, happen to many [k].

XIV. And to some indeed through whole Countries; from which Quarries of them have obtained their Names, as the *Parian*, the *Pentelican*, the *Chian*, and the *Theban* [l].

---

the Hiatus too large for that alone, have given their Opinion that the Word ἰδιότητας is also to be added in that Manner I have written it, and it appears evidently to me to have filled up a Gap in the Sense, as well as in the Writing, by making the Beginning, as well as all the rest of the Sentence, clearly refer to what I have observed the Author to have said before, Page 13 and of which this is no more than a Recapitulation in its proper Place

[k] The Author here gives an Account of the various Kinds of Marble and Alabaster known in his Time, and even so early as that, we find the *Parian* well known, and, as may very rationally be guessed from its being named before all the other Kinds, most esteemed of any. This was originally dug only in the Island of *Paros*, and the Strata of it were always found so cracked, that it is scarce ever to be had in Pieces of more than about five Feet long, so that the finest Blocks of it just served for Statues of a natural Size they were extremely valued for the Elegance of their Colour, and the excellent Polish they would take

A Marble of this Kind, but perhaps not exactly the same with this of the Ancients, is now dug in many Parts of *Italy*, and much esteemed for the same Qualities

The *Pentelican*, the Kind he next mentions, is now wholly unknown, and has been so for many Ages.

The *Chian* was a dark colour'd Marble formed from the Island of *Chios*, where it was dug, something of the Kind of

ιέ. Καὶ ὡς ὁ ἐν Αἰγύπτῳ περὶ Θήβας ἀλαβαςρίτης, ᾧ γὰρ ὄντῷ μέλας τέμνε]· ᾧ ὁ τῷ ἐλέφαντι
ὅμοιῷ, ὁ Χερνίτης καλύμΦ· ἐν ᾗ πυέλῳ φασὶ
ᾧ Δαρεῖον κεῖδς ᾧ ὁ πῶρῷ ὅμοιῷ τῷ χρώματι,
ᾧ τῇ πυκνότητι τῷ Παρίῳ, τὴ ϳ κεφότητα μόνον ἔχων
τῷ πώρῳ διὸ ᾧ ἐν τοῖς ἀνυδαζομένοις οἰκήμασιν,
ὥσπερ διάζαμα τιθέασιν αὐτὸν οἱ Αἰγύπτιοι

---

the Lapis Obsidianus of *Æthiopia*, and, like it, in some
Degree transparent

The *Theban* is a Marble well known to this Time, it
is red, variegated with other Colours, and is of two Kinds
The one softer, and marked only with yellow, which is
the *Brocatello* of the modern *Italians*, the other extremely
hard and variegated with Black, White, and many other
Colours This is the *Pyrrhopæcilus* and *Syenites* of *Pliny*,
and the *Granate* of the Moderns Many of the Works
of the Ancients in *Greece*, *Italy*, and elsewhere, are of this
Marble

The Alabaster is the *Alabastrites*, *Boet* 490 *De Lact*.
166. *Wirm* 42 *Matthiol* 1386 It is a well known
Stone, white, and approaching to the Nature of Marble,
but much softer The *Alabastrum* and *Alabastrites* of Naturalists, though by some esteemed synonymous Terms,
and by others confounded with one another, are different
Substances, the *Alabastrum* is properly the soft Stone, of a
gypseous Substance, burning easily into a Kind of Plaster;
and the *Alabastrites* the hard, bearing a good Polish, and
approaching to the Texture of Marble. All the later Authors confirm what *Theophrastus* here mentions, of its being found about *Thebes*. The Quarries of it there are not
yet exhausted, and probably will not be in many Ages.
This Stone was by the *Greeks* called also sometimes Onyx,
and by the *Latins*, *Marmor Onychites*, from its Use in
making Boxes for preserving precious Ointments, which
Boxes were commonly called Onyxes and Alabasters, Thus

(23)

XV In *Ægypt*, about *Thebes*, there is also found the *Alabaster*, which is dug in large Masses; and the *Chernites*, which resembles *Ivory*, and in which, it is said, *Darius* was buried, as also the *Porus*, which in Colour and Hardness emulates the *Parian* Marble, though singular in its remarkable Lightness, in which it resembles the *Tophus*, and on Account of which the *Ægyptians* generally used it in the Partitions of their more elegant Edifices

---

Dioscorides ἀλαβαστρίτη ὁ καλύμενος ὀνὺξ And hence have been a thousand Mistakes in the later Authors of less reading, who have misunderstood *Pliny*, and confounded the Onyx Marble, as the Alabaster was frequently called, with the precious Stone of that Name. This Author, however, cannot be accused of having given any Occasion to the Confusion, for though the Onyx was, in his Time, sometimes called also Alabaster, as well as the Alabaster Onyx, from their common Use in these Boxes, he here clearly explains himself as to which Kind he is treating of, by observing, that it is that which is dug in large Masses, by way of Distinction from the Onyx or Alabaster Gem, as what we now call only the Onyx was then sometimes called

The *Chernites*, or *Chernites*, was a white Marble, used in the Sepultures of the ancient *Greeks*, &c. and about which there have been many Mistakes among the later Authors, which, as the Species of Marble is now unknown among us, it would be but idle to enquire into

The *Porus* was also a Marble much in Esteem with the Ancients, but unknown to us. Its peculiar Property, as our Author observes, was its Lightness. It cut well, and bore a tolerable Polish, and the Statues, &c. made of it, were common in *Greece*, and called Πώρινα, as those of the Parian Marble were called Παρία. The *Tophus*, to which our Author compares this Marble for Lightness, is a rough Stone of the Pumice Kind, brittle, and easily crumbling into Powder. It is not much known in *England*, but common in *Germany*, where it is used instead of the Pumice, and called *Topffstein* and *Tugstein*. This was a Stone well

ιϛ'. Εὑρίσκε]) κὶ μέλας αὐτόθι διαφανὴς, ὁμοίως τῷ Χίῳ, κὶ παρ' ἄλλοις ἢ ἕτεροι πλείες.

ιζ'. Αἱ μ̃ ἓν τοιαῦ] διαφοραὶ, καθάπερ ἐλέχθη κοινότεραι πλείοσιν. αἱ δ κτ̃ τὰς δυνάμεις ᵐ τὰς προειρημένας, οὐκ ἔτι τοῖς ὅλοις ὑπάρχυσιν, ὐδὲ ζωο-

---

known among the *Greeks*, and was what they called the Porus, without any Addition, whereas the other, here described among the Marbles by the Author, was called the Porian Marble, from its Resemblance to this Porus. The dark transparent Stone, next mentioned, was probably of the Obsidianus Kind, as well as the Chian. The Antients had two or three of these dark Marbles, of fine Texture, in great Use among them. They bore a fine Polish, were transparent in some Degree when cut into thin Plates, and reflected the Images of Things as our Looking-glasses do the finest Kind was, for this Reason, called ὄψια ὃς ἀπὸ τῆς ὄψεως, which was afterwards written by the *Latins*, *Opsianus*, *Opsdianus*, and *Obsidianus*. And the true Origin of the Name being forgotten from the false spelling the Word, After-ages thought it had received it from one *Obsidius*, whom they imagined the first Finder of it.

ᵐ The Author, having now gone through the common Differences of the Strata of Stone, arising from common Causes, and particularly mentioned, and in few Words described the various Species of Marble known in his Time, comes now to the Consideration of certain more extraordinary Qualities in Stones of smaller Size, arising from the Powers of more particular Combinations of Matter in their Formation. The particular Stones he mentions in this Place, as possessing these Powers, are hereafter treated of more at large. I shall therefore refer, for what I have to observe in regard to them, to their proper Places, where they are separately described. To those particularly named the Author adds a great Number, which he also hereafter describes, in the Words τῶν εἰς τὰ σφραγίδια γλυπτῶν, which I have chosen to translate " that are cut as Gems,"

XVI There is also found in the same Place a transparent *Stone*, something like the *Chian*, and in others, there are many other Kinds.

XVII These then are the Differences which have been mentioned as common to many *Stones*. But those which arise from the particular Powers [m] before named, are less frequent; nor do they, like these,

---

not as the literal Meaning of the Words might seem to imply, limiting what are added only to those on which Seals were engraven. It is evident, the Author meant himself no such Limitation, since he has afterwards described, among the Stones of this Class, many which he expressly says were too small for this particular Use. The Reason of his using that Word in this Place is, that the *Greeks* had no particular Name for the pellucid Stones, which we call distinctly Gems, they called all Stones, whether large or small, hard or soft, precious or common, by the general Name λίθος, and distinguished them, one from another, by their Epithets only, as διαφανὴς &c and as the general Use of what we call Gems, and they had no particular Name for, was the serving for Seals, they sometimes, instead of distinguishing them by particular or descriptive Epithets, called them Seal Stones, and hence the Word Seal Stone σφραγὶς, or σφραγιδίου became with them a common Word for what we call Gem, and in that Sense it is evidently used here by this Author.

Most of the Stones of this Class were found to be of so compact a Texture, as to resist the Force of Fire, at least of common Fires, and even the strongest known in this Author's Time; the solar indeed, which we are able to throw on Bodies, by reflecting Burning-glasses, no Stone, not even the Diamond, in all Circumstances and Positions, can withstand. But as some Stones, which he had yet to treat of, were subject to great Changes, from the Action of Fire, such as was then commonly used on certain Occasions, whether culinary, or for the melting of Metals, these he first chuses to describe, and proceeds to give the several Differences of,

ἐχείαις λίθων, οὐδὲ μεγέθεσιν· ἔνιοι δὴ καὶ σπάνιοι
πάμπαν εἰσὶ καὶ σμικροὶ, καθάπερ ἥ τε, σμάραγδος,
καὶ τὸ σάρδιον, καὶ ὁ ἄνθραξ, καὶ ἡ σάπφειρος, καὶ
σχεδὸν λόγῳ τῶν εἰς τὰ σφραγίδια γλυπτῶν. οἱ δὲ ἐν
ἑτέροις εὑρίσκονται διακοπτομένοις.

ιά. Ὀλίγοι δὲ καὶ οἱ περὶ τὴν πύρωσιν, καὶ καῦσιν.
ὑπὲρ ὧν δὴ καὶ πρῶτον ἴσως λεκτέον, τίνας καὶ πόσας
ἔχουσιν διαφορὰς.

ιβ΄. Κατὰ δὴ τὴν πύρωσιν οἱ μὲν τήκονται καὶ ῥέουσιν,
ὥσπερ οἱ μεταλλωτοί· ῥεῖ γὰρ ἅμα τῷ ἀργύρῳ, καὶ τῷ
χαλκῷ καὶ σιδήρῳ [n] καὶ ἡ λίθος ἡ ἐκ τούτων. εἰ τοίνυν
διὰ τὴν ὑγρότητα τῶν ὑπαρχόντων, εἴτε καὶ δι' αὐτάς.
ὡσαύτως δὲ καὶ οἱ πυρομάχοι, καὶ οἱ μυλίαι ῥέουσιν, οἷς
ἐπιτιθέασιν οἱ καίοντες.

---

[n] The Author is here treating of the various Kinds of *Spars*, formed near the Veins of different Metals, and assuming their Colours from, and partaking of the Natures of the particular Metals in the Mines or which they are found. All these are formed by the Percolation and Afflux of their constituent Matter, which is taken up by the Water continually pervading the Strata, and in its Way separated from the grosser Particles it was at first reposited among, and mixed with, and finally tinged with a Colour from, and in some Degree impregnated with the Virtues of the metalline Matter, among which it is deserted by the Water in which it was before suspended, and left to coagulate, and assume the Form naturally arising from the Concretion of its Parts. Where these Spars are formed out of the Reach of metalline Matter, and have received, in their Passage through the Strata, no Impregnations from

happen to whole Strata, or vaſt Maſſes: Some of the Stones, in which they take Place, are very ſcarce and ſmall, as the *Emerald*, the *Carnelian*, the *Carbuncle*, the *Sapphire*, and, in general, all that are cut as *Gems*; and ſome of them are found in dividing other Stones.

XVIII. Some few of theſe Stones there are, which are ſubject to the Force of *Fire*, and may be burnt. Theſe ſhall be firſt treated of, in Conſideration of what their Differences are.

XIX. In regard to the Action of Fire on them, ſome are *fuſible*, and melt by it, as the metalline Kinds. For the *Stones*, which partake of the Nature of *Metals*, as *Silver*, *Copper*, or *Iron*, [n] melt in the Furnaces with them, either by means of the Humidity of the metalline Matter they partake of, or of their own Nature. And in this Manner the *Pyritæ* also, and thoſe Kinds of them called the *Molares*, melt with the Matter they are laid on in burning [n].

---

it, they are white, which is the natural Colour of their conſtituent Particles, but where they are formed in or about Mines, they, as our Author very juſtly remarks, partake of the Nature of, and, in ſome Degree, owe their Form and Mode of Exiſtence to the particular Metal of the Mine. Their Shape and Virtues are often given them by the metalline Particles mixed with them in their Concretions, their Colours always, and that in a ſtronger or fainter Degree, as there has been more or leſs of that Matter mingled in their Maſſes.

If the metalline Particles are in the Mixture in any conſiderable Quantity, the whole aſſumes a Shape peculiar to the Metal to which they belong, if that be *Lead*, the ſparry Concretions are cubic; if *Iron*, rhomboidal; and if *Tin*, they ſhoot into the Form of quadralateral Pyramids. Theſe are the Metals of which we can pretty certainly

κ'. Οἱ ὃ κ̀ ὅλως λέγϫσι πάν]ας τήκεϑ̓, πλὼ
ϛ̃ μαρμάρϫ. τϫ́τον ὃ καΤακαίεϑ̓, κ̀ κονίαν ἐξ
αυτϋ γίνεϑαι. δόξειε δ' ἂν ϫ́τως ὅλως ἐπὶ πλεῖον
εἰρῆϑ̓.

---

judge, from the Figure of the Spar about the Mine, for the others, though they influence the shooting of it in no less Degree, yet they do not always throw it into such determinate or regular Figures

But if the metalline Particles, assumed into the Spar at the Time of its Concretion, have a very great Power in determining it to a certain Figure, the Influence they have over it, in regard to Colour, is much greater, as all that it has of that is wholly owing to them, and as they are in greater or lesser Quantities in it, they give it different Degrees of it, from the slightest Tinge to the deepest Colour.

What Metal has been concerned in effecting this Change of Colour, is not less easily and certainly discoverable from the Colour itself, than what has influenced the Shape, from the Shape. If *Lead* has furnished the metalline Particles, the Spar is yellow, if *Iron*, red, if *Tin*, black, if *Copper*, it is either greenish or bluish, according to the Quality of the Menstruum Nature has furnished for dissolving the Particles of that Metal, and bringing them into a State of mixing in the Concretion, for Acids and Alkalis both dissolve Copper, but with this Difference of Colour, that the Solution with an Acid is green, and that with an Alkali is blue.

Though this Author was perfectly right, therefore, in his Opinion of these Substances partaking of the Nature of the Metals they were found among; he errs in imagining that they are fusible, and melt with those Metals, he may very well, however, be pardoned in this, since it has been an Error which many later Authors, who had more Opportunities of informing themselves of the Truth than he can reasonably be supposed to have had, have also fallen into, nay, and many who imagine they understand these Things very well, from the constant Use of it in fluxing

XX. Some absolutety affirm, that all *Stones* will melt in the Fire except *Marble*, which by burning is reduced to Ashes: But this is saying absolutely, and of all, what ought only to be said in general, and of the greater Number.

---

the Ores of Metals, believe the same of it even yet. This is however an absolutely erroneous Opinion, for Spar is not fusible, but calcines in the Fires used for melting the Ores of Metals. The Use it is of, in the fusing them is this. Those Ores are frequently clogged and loaded with Sulphurs, which make them very difficult of Fusion; and the Calx of Spar is of the same Use in that Case, that Lime, or any other fixed Alkali would be; that is, it absorbs those Sulphurs, and by that means destroying what would impede the Fusion of the Ore, does in some Sense assist its melting; but no one, who ever saw the Fusion of Ore with its Spar about it, ever yet observed the least Particle of that to melt.

The Pyritæ and Molares, as many Kinds of them were originally called, are no more capable of Fusion in the Fire than the Spars. They are Masses of mineral, saline, and sulphureous Matter, either in detached Pieces of different Figures and Textures, or in whole Veins. The various Kinds of them contain different Quantities of different Metals, but generally too small to be worth the Charge and Trouble of working. Gold, Silver, Copper, and Iron are frequently found thus in them. But the principal Substances of which they are formed are Salts, Sulphurs, and Earths. The common Copperas of our Shops is made from different Kinds of them, in different Quantities, and no Species yields it in such Plenty as the echinated Kind of the Chalk Pits of *Kent* and *Surrey*. The Marchasites, as those are particularly called which are not in detached Pieces, but run in Veins, or fill the perpendicular Fissures of Strata, often abound with Copper, and with a mineral, arsenical Juice, seldom found in the others; some of these also contain Antimony, others Bismuth, and some Iron and Tin. When they are very rich in these Metals, they lose the Name of Marchasites, and are

κά. Πολλοὶ γὰ οἱ ῥηγνύμενοι° κỳ διαπηδῶντες ὡς, ἐ μαχίμενοι (κζ´) τ̄ πυρώσιν, ὥσπερ ὐδὲ ὁ κέραμ(ο). ὁ κỳ κζ´ λόγον ἐςίν. οἵ τινες ἐξυιρασμένοι τυγχάνυσιν. τὸ γὰ τηκτὸν, ἔνικμον εἶναι ἀεὶ, καὶ ὑγρότητα ἔχι πλείω.

---

called Ores. The Mineral, called in some Parts of *England* *Mundick*, is of this Kind, containing Copper and sometimes other Metals; but the Sulphur is so abundant in these Kinds of Ores, that they are not to be fluxed without great Trouble, the Addition of Lime, or some similar Substance, is often necessary to bring them to fuse it all, and at best they are the most troublesome, and least profitable, unless where very rich indeed, of any Ores in the World.

This Author however was not single, though erroneous, in his Opinion of the Pyritæ and Molares melting in the Fire; his Master *Aristotle* had probably led him into it, who has, Met. L. 4. c. 6. τήκεται δὲ κỳ ὁ λίθ᾽, ὁ πυρίμαχος ὥστε ῥεῖν κ ῥεῖν, τὸ δὲ πηλῶδεσον ὅταν ξηρανθῇ πάλιν γίνεται σκληρὸς, κỳ αἱ μυλίαι τήκονται ὥστε ῥεῖν.

° Some few Species of Flints are Substances of this Kind, and above all others that found in whole Strata (not in detached Masses or Nodules, as the common Flints are) and called *Chert* or *Whern* in some Parts of *England*, a Lump of this, put into a moderate Fire, will, as the Heat penetrates it, fly to Pieces in Scales or thin Flakes, which fall off, from Time to Time, till the whole is reduced to a Mass of coarse Powder, but it is an Error to infer from this, that these Stones are not fusible, for the same Stone, or even the very Powder, into which it has been shattered by the Fire, put into a Crucible with Salt of Tartar, or any other fixed alkaline Salt, and placed in a stronger Fire, will melt and boil in the Vessel, and form a very good Glass, as I have many Times experienced.

XXI. For some burst° and fly in Pieces in the Fire, as, though not fusible, yet not of Power wholly to resist the Force of the Heat; which is also the Case in earthen Vessels: And this is an Effect no way repugnant to Reason; for these are absolutely dry, whereas whatever is fusible must be, at least in some Degree, moist, and retain, to the Time of its Fusion, more or less of its Humidity.

To learn the real Causes of the different Degrees of this Fusibility in different fossile Substances, it will be necessary, first, to consider the Cause of their Solidity, or, in other Words, of their Cohesion, and this, as I have before observed, is that Power residing in all Matter, called Attraction.

This Power, it has also already been observed, is infinitely strongest at the Point of Contact, and therefore the Cohesion of all Bodies must be in Proportion to the Number of Points in which their constituent Particles touch one another. Those Particles therefore which have the least Solidity, with relation to their Surfaces, though they attract least at Distances, yet, when they touch, cohere the most intimately; but where, from contrary Causes, the Cohesion is small, as in spherical Bodies, whose Surfaces can only touch in a Point, their Particles easily recede from one another on any Impulse, and whenever they are set in Motion, Fluidity takes Place.

By what means Fire is an Agent in bringing Things into this State, is easily understood. Its Particles, which are very powerful and very active, insinuate themselves into the Substance of the Matter to be melted, break and divide its Particles, and occasion a much smaller Contact of Parts than there was before, and of course a weaker Cohesion, more fiery Particles continually getting in as the Matter continues on the Fire, more and more diminish the Degree of Contact, till at last there is not enough of it to keep the Particles from rolling one over another, that is coming into a State of Fusion.

(32)

κϛ′. Φασὶ δὲ κὶ τ̄ ἡλιγμένων τὰς μὲν ἀναξηραίνεσθαι τελείως, ὥς᾽ ἀχρείας εἶναι μὴ καταβρεχθέντας πάλιν καὶ ζυνικμασθέντας τὰς δὲ κὶ μαλακωτέρας ϗ διαθραύςτας μᾶλλον. Φανερὸν δὲ ὡς ἀμφοτέρων μὲν ἐξαιρεῖςθ τ̄ ὑγρότητα. Συμβαίνει δὲ τὰς μ̄ πυκνὰς ἀποξηραινομένας σκληρύνεςθ· τὰς δὲ μανὰς, κὶ ὧν ἡ φύσις τοιαύτη, θραυσὰς εἶναι ϗ τηκτὰς.

κγ′. Ἔνιοι δὲ τ̄ θραυσῶν ἀνθρακοῦντ] τῇ καύσει, κὶ διαμένυσι πλείω χρόνον. ὥσπερ οἱ περὶ Βίνας ἐν τῷ μετάλλῳ κὶ ὃς ὁ ποταμὸς καταφέρει. καίον] γὸ ὅταν ἄνθρακες ἐπιτεθῶσι, ϗ μέχρι τέτυ χρείας ἐὰν φυσᾷ τις εἶτ᾽ ἀπομαραίνοντ], κὶ πάλιν καίοντ]. διὸ κὶ πολὺν χρόνον ἡ χρῆσις. ἡ δ᾽ ὀσμὴ βαρεῖα σφόδρα κὶ δυχερής [p].

This is the general Cause of the Fusion of fossile and other Substances, and the different Degrees of Fire, they require to bring them to it, are proportioned to their different Contact of Parts or Degrees of Cohesion; such as have least Contacts melt soonest, and for this Reason Lead melts more readily than Gold the different Gravity of the Substances has nothing to do in this, since it is not according to the Quantity of Matter they contain, but the Number of Points in which the Particles of that Matter touch one another, and for this Reason it is that Lead, which is heavier than most other Metals, notwithstanding its superior Quantity of Matter, melts also more readily than most others

[p] The Stone here described is the Lapis Thracius of the

later

XXII. It is said also, that on exposing to the Sun's Rays some are wholly dried up, so as to be rendered useless, unless macerated and impregnated again with Moisture; while others, by the same means become softer and more brittle. It is evident that the Humidity is extracted in both these Cases; the Difference is, that the more dense and compact harden by this drying; whereas the looser, and those of a less firm Texture, become more brittle and soft by it.

XXIII. Some of the more brittle *Stones* there also are, which become as it were burning Coals, when put into a Fire, and continue so a long time; of this Kind are those about *Bena*, found in Mines, and wash'd down by the Torrents, for they will take fire on throwing burning Coals on them, and continue burning so long as any one blows them; afterwards they will deaden, and may after that be made to burn again. They are therefore of long Continuance, but their Smell is troublesome and disagreeable P,

---

later Authors, a Stone much talked of in all the Writings of the Naturalists, and by some allowed a Place in the Catalogues of the *Materia Medica*, but now wholly unknown. There is, however, no question, from our Author's Account of this Substance, but that it was the very Thing afterwards well known under that Name. *Bina*, or *Bena*, the Place he mentions where it was found, was a Town in *Thracia*, and every Particular he has recorded of it has been since applied to the *Lapis Thracius*. It's inflammable Quality, disagreeable Smell, and the Manner in which it was found, were the same with those of the *Thracius* of the later Writers. This was well known to *Dioscorides*, &c. as is evident from what they have said of it, but there has been so much Confusion about it among the

D

κδ'. Ὃν ἢ καλῦσι σπίνον, ὡς ἦν ἐν τοῖς μετάλλοις, τοιῦτος διακοπεὶς ἢ ζωπυρηθεὶς πρὸς ἑαυτὸν, ἐν τῷ ἡλίῳ τιθέμεν@, καίε], ἢ μᾶλλον ἐὰν ἐπιψεκάζῃ, ἢ πυράνη τις ᵠ.

Writers since, that little more than the Name has been handed down to us, some have been of opinion, that it was a kind of *Coal*, others of *Jet*, and others of the *Ampelitis*. What is to be gathered from the Antients about it is, that it was a hard bituminous Substance, very inflammable, of a brittle Texture, and of a very disagreeable Smell when burning. It was sometimes dug, as our Author observes, but principally found in the River *Pontus*, into which it had probably been washed from the Banks, in the Strata of which it was originally lodged, by the dashing of the waves in Storms, or dislodged by other Accidents. As is also the Case with the *Pyritæ*, *Ludus Helmontii*, Amber, and many other of the fossile Substances, which are now generally found on the Shores of the Sea or large Rivers, and of which a diligent Enquirer will always find a much larger Quantity in the Strata of the neighbouring Land, than are seen washed on the Shore, and generally many standing out from among the Matter of the Strata of the Shores or adjacent Cliffs, and ready to be washed out by Rains, or dislodged by the Earth of the Strata cracking after Frost, and so rolled down into the River, tho' in their natural Situation out of the reach of its Waves, the dashing of which in Storms and high Tides against the Banks, are the more common Means of getting them out.

Most of the Editions have it ἀδεκπυρῦναι τῇ ξηρασία, *Salmasius* first restored the Passage to its original Sense, by altering it to τῇ καύσει, which there is no room to doubt was the original Reading. Nor is that the only Thing in which this Sentence is indebted to that excellent Critick for restoring it to its native Sense and Purity, as indeed are many other Parts of this Author's Works.

ᵠ The *Spinus*, or, as the excellent Critic just mentioned would have it called, *Spilus*, σπῖλος, was another in-

XXIV. That also which is called the *Spinus*, is found in Mines. This Stone cut in Pieces and thrown together in a Heap, exposed to the Sun, burns, and that the more, if it be moistened or sprinkled with Water [a].

---

doubted Bitumen of the *Iapis Thracius* Kind, of which *Theophrastus* is not the only Author who has recorded this memorable Quality, which we have no Right either to confirm or question, as the Substance is now wholly unknown to us.

The general Characteristics of these solid Bitumens, the Class of Bodies the Author is here describing, are, that they are dense, dry, and friable Substances, easily inflammable, fusible by Fire, and condensing by Cold. They are soluble in Oil, not to be disunited by Water, as the igniceous Earths are, and yield in Distillation a large Quantity of fetid Oil.

The Bodies of this Class, known to the Antients and understood under this general Name, were, beside the *Thracius* and *Spinus*, 1. The *Asphaltum*, called also *Bitumen Judaicum*, and by *Serapion*, *Gummi funerum*, this was found in *Dioscorides*'s Time about *Sidon* in *Phœnicia*, *Zait* in *Sicily*, and in *Judæa*. The Account in the sacred Writings, of its having been used as Mortar in the building the Tower of *Babel*, is unquestionable; *Strabo* and others of the Antients asserting, that it was found plentifully about *Babylon*, and that the Buildings of the old *Babylon* were of Brick cemented with this Substance.

2. The *Pissasphaltos*, found, according to *Dioscorides*, in the Ceraunian Mountains of *Apollonia*; this was not so hard as the former, and of a more pleasant Smell; it is now found in the Campania of *Rome*, near a small Town called *Catho*, where it ouzes through the Crannies of Rocks, and is at first of the Consistence of Honey, but soon dries and becomes hard.

3. Amber, of which the Author treats hereafter in this Work.

4. Jet, the *Gagates* of *Dioscorides*, and black Amber of the Shops, a dry, hard, shining Substance, of a fine

κί. Ὁ δὲ Λιπαραῖος r ἐκπυροῦται τῇ καύσει, καὶ γίνεται κισσηροειδής ὥσθ' ἅμα τὴν τε χρόαν μεταβάλλειν καὶ τὴν πυκνότητα. μέλας τε γὰρ καὶ λεῖος ἐστι, καὶ πυκνός, ἄκαυστος ὤν γίνεται δ' ὅτ(αν) ἐν τῇ κισ-

---

black, burning like Pitch, and emitting a thick black Smoke. Its Name it had from *Gagis*, a Town in *Lycia*, where it was originally found, it is now dug in *France*, *Germany*, *Savoy*, and some Parts of *England*.

5. Cannel Coal, the Ampelites of *Dioscorides*, called its *Terra Ampelitis* by some Authors, tho' its Use in Medicine at present is almost wholly unknown. This is harder than the foregoing, and takes an excellent Polish, we have it in many Parts of *Ireland*, where it is turned into Toys of many Kinds. And

6. The Lithanthrax, or common Coal, well known to all.

These were the solid Bitumens, known as such to the Antients, and since tho' they were not all known so early as in this Author's Days, I judged it not amiss thus shortly to mention here, that it may be observed from their Characters and Descriptions, and those of the two mentioned by the Author, that it was neither of these that he knew by either of the two Names of those he has described.

The *Lipara* Stone (so called from *Lipare*, one of the Æolian Islands, from whence it was usually brought among the Pumices of which those Islands always furnished a large Quantity) is a small Stone, usually about the bigness of a Filbert, of an irregular and uncertain Shape, and porous friable Constitution, like that of the Pumices, but more easily crumbling to Powder between the Fingers than even the softest Kinds of them. The Colour is generally of a dusky grey, and the whole external Face of it evidently shews that it has suffered Changes by the Fire. The Antients had these Stones in great Esteem, and *Pliny* has recorded an idle Tradition concerning them, which I suppose was then generally believed, *suffita ea omnes bestias evocari*, but at present they are so little regarded, that

XXV. *But the *Lipara* Stone empties itself as it were in burning, and becomes like the *Pumice*, changing at once both its Colour and Density, for before burning it is black, smooth, and compact. This Stone is found in the *Pumices*, separately, in different

---

the Writers on these Subjects have even forgot to name them, and *Worm*, the only Naturalist of (...) ones, who had actually received them, and give them a Place in his Museum, and a Description in the History of it, seems not to have known that it ever had any Name at all. I don't know that any body else has observed that his *lapilli cinerei Ftnæ*, are the *Lapides* or *Liparaus Lapis* of the Antients, but his Description so exactly agrees with some Stones I have, which I received with some Pumice from *Ætna*, and have always judged to be the *Liparas*, that I make not the least question of their being the very Sorts. His Words are, *Ejusdam montis (sc. Ætnæ) ei ab (...) ejecta, ad nos delati sunt Lapilli, cinerei, obscuri & adusti, qui vi ignis naturam fuam plane amiserunt, et pene sui reddid, laxes & inæquales, ita ut ad naturam Pumicum quam proxime accedant, sed friabiliores sint & facile in minutores partes, vel digitorum compressi diffluant.*

Besides those which I have from *Ætna*, I have sometimes seen of them among Quantities of Pumice. I cannot say I ever had the Fortune to find any one in a Mass of the Pumice, or ever had an Opportunity of observing their Texture before they had passed the Fire, but the Account this Author gives of them may probably enough be true in both Circumstances, it being very common to observe fresh Stones of the Flint, Pebble, and other kind, immersed in Masses of a different Texture; and the intense Degree of Heat these, with the Pumices, must have suffered, might very probably effect Changes as great or much greater, than between the present State of this Stone and what this Author describes to have been its Original.

As to what regards the Pumice itself, as the Author hereafter describes it more at large, I shall reserve to that Place what I have to observe about it.

σήρα διειλημμβύ@. ἄλλοθι κ ἄλλοθι, καθάπερ ἐν κυ-
ταρείω, κ ὐ ζωνεχής· ὥσπερ κ ἐν Μήλῳ φασὶ τὼ
κίστηραν ἐν ἄλλῳ τινὶ λίθῳ γίνεοζ κ ἐκεῖν@ μ
τύτῳ ὥσπερ ἀντιπεπονθώς. πλὼ ὁ λίθος ὗτος ὀκ
ὁμοι@ τῷ Λιπαραίῳ.

κϛ'. Ἐκπυρῦται δὲ κ ὁ ἐν Τεργεδὶ τῆς Σικελίας
γινόμβν@. τῦτο δὲ τὸ χωρίον ἐστὶ κατ Λιπάρην.

κζ'. Ὁ δὲ λίθ@ ἐν τῇ ἄκρᾳ τῇ Ἐρνεάδι καλυ-
μβύη πολὺς, ὁμοίως τ̄ Βινας καιόμβν@, ὀσμὼ
ἀφίησιν ἀσφάλζ. τὸ δ' ἐκ τῆς κατακαύσεως ὅμοιον
γίνεζ γῇ κεκαυμβύη.

κη'. Οὓς δὲ καλῦσιν ἐυθὺς ἄνθρακας, τ̄ θρυπτο-
μβύων διὰ τὼ χρείαν, εἰσι γεώδεις. ἐκκαίονζ δὲ κ
πυρῦνζ καθάπερ οἱ ἄνθρακες. εἰσὶ δὲ περί τε τὼ
Λιγυστικὼ, ὅπυ κὴ τὸ ἤλεκζον, κ ἐν τῇ Ἠλείᾳ,
βαδιζόντων Ὀλυμπιάζε τὼ δ' ὄρυς. οἷς κ οἱ χαλ-
κεῖς χρῶνζ ᵗ.

ᵇ The Name of this Place is differently spelt in different
Editions of this Author, some having it Τηρα, others
Τελαρία, and probably neither of them right, for there is
no mention of any Place in Sicily of either the one or the
other of these Names in the antient Geography. But
however uncertain the Place of Production of these Stones
be, what our Author observes of them is very well worth
noting, that they become light, porous, and resembling
Pumices from the Action of the Fire. It were much to
be wish'd we were now acquainted with this Stone, since
if we knew any which we could by Fire reduce to a Pumice, it would give us a Light into the Origin of that
Body, which we at present very much want.

The Substance next mentioned is evidently of the Class
of solid Bitumens, and a Species of the *Lapis Thracius*

Places, and as it were in Cells, no where continuous to the Matter of them. It is said, that in *Melos* the Pumice is produced in this Manner in some other Stone, as this is on the contrary in it. But the Stone which the Pumice is found in is not at all like the *Lipara* Stone, which is found in it.

XXVI. Certain Stones there are about *Tetras* in *Sicily*, which is over against *Lipara*, which empty themselves in the same manner in the Fire.

XXVII. And in the Pomontory called *Erineas*, there is a great Quantity of Stone like that found about *Bena*, which, when burnt, emits a bituminous Smell, and leaves a Matter resembling calcined Earth.

XXVIII. Those fossile Substances that are called Coals, and are broken for Use, are earthy, they kindle however, and burn like wood Coals. These are found in *Liguria*, where there also is Amber, and in *Elis*, in the Way to *Olympics* over the Mountains. These are used by the Smiths[†]

---

before described. The Residuum after burning, or *Caput* of all the Bitumens, is a calcined Earth, and Rocks and Promontories are the most common Places out of which they are found exsudating.

[†] The Substance here described, whatever Mistakes there have been among Authors since about it, appears to me to be evidently no other than the common Pit Coal, and I have made it appear so clearly so in the Translation, only by having properly rendered the Word ἄνθραξ, the careless misunderstanding which Word alone has been the Occasion of all the erroneous Guesses about the Substance here described. The Authors of these seem all to have understood the Word ἄνθραξ, as signifying Fossile or Pit Coal, and therefore, as the Author compares the burning of this Substance to that, they were necessitated to think of

(40)

κθ´. Εὑρέθη δέ ποτε ᵛ ἐν (τοῖς) Σκαπτησύλης μετάλλοις λίθος, ὃς τῇ μ̅ ὄψει παρόμοιος ὢν ξύλῳ σαπρῷ· ὅτε δ᾽ ἐπιχέοιτό τις ἔλαιον, καίεται· κ̀ ὅτ᾽ ἐκκαυθείη, τότε παύεται κ̀ αὐτὸς, ὥσπερ ἀπαθὴς ὤν.

λ´. Τῶν μ̅ ἐν καιομένων αὗται διαφοραί.

λά. Ἄλλο δέ τι γένος ἐστὶ λίθων, ὥσπερ ἐξ ἐναντίων πεφυκός, ἄκαυστον ʷ ὅλως, ˣ ἄνθραξ καλύμενος.

---

some other Substance that he might here mean, as it was impossible he should intend to compare a Thing to itself.

Kentius, on this Foundation, imagined, that he meant the Cannel Coal. *Quod Galenus vocat Phidentidem, & Theophrastus Carbones vocat quod eorum colorem habeat, & vices gerat.* Thus is *Theophrastus*, according to Custom, accused of saying Things he never meant, because the People who quote him have not been at the pains to understand him. ἐκκαίεται δὲ κ̀ ὥσπερ ξύλα καίονται οἱ ἄνθρακες, is evidently, they kindle and burn like Wood Coals, or, as we call it, Charcoal, for that is the genuine and determinate Sense of the Word ἄνθραξ in *Greek*, and *Carbo* in *Latin*, as is evident from the other Works of this Author, *Pliny*, and all the other old Naturalists, and even the more correct of the Moderns, when they would express what we call Pit Coal, the Substance here described by the Author, never use the Words ἄνθραξ or *Carbo* alone, but always *Carbo fossilis*, and λιθάνθραξ. See *Woodward*, *Charlton*, *Merret*, &c. The similar Use of this Bitumen got it the Name of Coal, but always with an Addition that distinguished it from what was more commonly and properly so called, and expressed its not being of vegetable, but fossile Origin.

ᵛ It is much to be questioned, whether this was the true original Reading, and genuine Sense of the Author, in all probability some Errors in the old Editions have made this

XXIX. There is also found in the Mines of *Scaptesylæ* a Stone, in its external Appearance something resembling rotten Wood, on which, if Oil be poured, it burns; but when the Oil is burnt away, the burning of the Stone ceases, as if it were in itself not liable to such Accidents.

XXX. These then are the Differences of the Stones which are subject to the Force of Fire.

XXXI. But there is another Kind of Stone, formed, as it were, of contrary Principles, and entirely incombustible [w], which is called the [x] Car-

---

Passage express what the Author never meant to say. The Substance, and indeed the only Substance described by the other antient Naturalists, as resembling rotten Wood, is the Gagates or Jet before mentioned among the Bitumens, but that has no such Quality as the Author has here ascribed to this Stone of *Scaptesylæ*.

The Antients, it is to be observed, had a common Opinion of the Bitumens, that the Fire of them was encreased by Water, and extinguished by Oil; and very probably this was the Sentiment originally delivered here by the Author, however Errors upon Errors in different Copies of his Works may since have altered the Sense of them. The Stone itself was probably a Bitumen of the *Lapis Thracius* Kind, as the Place from whence it hath its Name was a Town of that Country.

[w] The Author having now gone through the different Effects of Fire on the different Kinds of Stones which are subject to be acted upon by it, comes here to the Consideration of some others, which, either from the different Matter of their constituent Particles, or the different Manner of their Combinations, he esteems of a Texture not to be injured by Fire, but altogether safe against its Efforts, and, as his own Words express it, incombustible.

None of these indeed are of Power to resist the solar Fire collected by a great reflecting Burning-glass, but are first calcined as it were, and split and shattered in Pieces

ἐξ οὗ καὶ τὰ σφραγίδια γλύφουσιν. ἐρυθρὸν μ̃ τῷ χρώ-

---

by it, and afterwards melted into a Glass. This, however, was probably a kind of Fire unknown in these extreme Degrees of Power, till very long since the Time of this Author. And as the culinary Fire, or that used in those Times for fluxing Ores, the strongest they then knew, tho' much less intense than those we now use on that Occasion (of which there are many unquestionable Proofs; nay, that even those of the Workers in Metals, but a few Ages ago were so) had no Power of making any Change in these Stones, the Author is not to be censured for esteeming them incombustible, or not knowing what it was impossible he should have seen, but is to be understood with regard to the Action of the Fires used in his time, and must then be allowed to have been well acquainted with the Subjects he treats of in this Division of his Work.

x The Antients expressed by this Word all the red transparent Gems, which have been since distinguished under the Names of the different Kinds of Ruby, Granate, Hyacynth, &c. all which they esteemed only different Species of the Carbuncle. And in Justification of them it must be acknowledged, that not only the fossile Genera in general want those fixt and determinate Characteristics, by which those of the vegetable and animal Kingdoms are unalterably distinguished from each other, but that those of the Gems in particular have fewer fixed and unvariable Differences by which their Genera and Species may be determinately fixed, than any other.

The Reason of the Difficulty in regularly methodizing and distinguishing the Genera and subordinate Species in the various Classes of the fossile Kingdom, is, that in the Time of their original Concretions their Particles scarce ever coalesced in perfect Purity, but took up among them from amidst the Mass of fluid Matter in which they were at that Time sustained, Particles of extraneous Matter of various Kinds in various Places; so that not only the external Face, but even the interior Constitution of the same Species is found in different Places very different, and in

buncle, on which they engrave Seals. Its Colour is red, and of such a Kind, that when held against

---

many Specimens not to be known at first sight even to the most accurate Observer.

But if this be the Case in fossile Substances in general, it is much more particularly so in this Class of them, the Gems, the Differences of which are owing to the Distribution of certain kind of Particles in their Masses, which are so very uncertain, both in Quantity and Manner of placing, and in their various Effects upon the Mass, that scarce any thing of certainty is to be determined from them.

What can be ascertained in general is this.

The Mass of constituent Matter of them all, is a pellucid crystalline Substance, which is in different Kinds of different Degrees of Hardness, from that of the Diamond to that of the merest shattery Crystal. This crystalline Matter, had it concreted in perfect Purity, had been colourless alike in all, and the various Species had been distinguishable only by their different Degrees of Hardness; but as this Matter, in the time of its Coalescence, assumed into it any Particles of a proper degree of Gravity and Fineness, which happened to float in its Way, it became by that Means different not only in Colour, nay, and in Degree of Colour, according to the Nature and Quantity of the Particles it took up into itself, but from their different Nature was also altered in what alone could have been its determinate Characteristics, its Hardness and Specifick Gravity. Many Reasons may be alledged that the Particles thus assumed into the crystalline Nodules at the Time of their Formation, must have been principally of the metalline Kind, and we find, in effect, that it was so. The various Colours of the Gems have their Rise from these Admixtures, and, according to what I have before observed as to the colouring of Spars by the same Means, when the metalline Matter thus mixed with the crystalline was Lead, the Stone became a Topaz, or, as the Antients call'd it, a Chrysolite, for it is very evident, that what they call'd the Topaz, we now call the Chrysolite, and what they call'd the Chrysolite, we now, on the contrary, call the Topaz.

μαῖι, πρὸς ϳ τ᾿ ᾿ ἥλιον τιθέμλνον, ἄνθρακος καιομῄ
ποιεῖ χρέαν Τιμιώτατον δ᾿ ὡς εἰπεῖν. μικρον γὰρ
σφόδρα, τεἸραρκονῖα χρυσῶν. ἄγεϳ δ᾿ ἔτ@ ἐκ
Καρχηδόν@ ἓ Μασσαλίας

λϛ´. Οὐ καίεϳ δ᾿ ὁ περὶ Μίλητον ᵘ γωνιειδὴς ὤν.

Our Topaz is a very elegant and very beautiful Gem, of which the Jewellers have two Kinds, the Oriental and Occidental, the Oriental are of a fine pure gold Colour, of different Degrees of Deepness. They are of very great Splendour, and equal the Ruby in Hardness. They are brought from *Arabia*, and many Parts of the *East Indies*. The Occidental are often very beautiful, and scarce to be distinguished from the Oriental but by their Softness, for they are no harder than common Crystal. We have them from *Silesia* and *Bohemia*.

The Topaz of the Antients, now call'd the Chrysolite, differs from this in Colour, for it has always an Admixture of green with the yellow, probably from Particles of Copper dissolved in an Acid, and taken up with those of the Lead into the Matter of the Gem, at the Time of its original Concretion.

As these Gems have their Colours from this accidental Admixture of extraneous Particles, they may also be divested of them by Fire, without any Injury to their Texture, and the Oriental Topaz thus rendered colourless, is like some other Gems to be hereafter described, sometimes made to counterfeit a Diamond.

When Lead and Iron together thus entred the Composition, the Stone became a Hyacynth, when Iron alone, the Ruby Granate, and other red Gems, or, as the Antients in one Word express it, the Carbuncles were produced, when Copper, dissolved by Acids, the Emerald, by Alcalies, the Sapphire, and so of the rest. No Wonder is it, therefore, that the Gems in particular have never been perfectly reduced to Method, since there is so little Room for determining any thing fix'd and stable in regard to them, and when the Operations by which Nature gave them their Existence, have been so uncertain and liable to such numberless accidental Variations.

the [y] Sun, it resembles that of a burning Coal. This Stone is extremely valuable, one of a very small Size being prized at forty Aurei. It is brought from *Carthage* and *Massilia*.

XXXII. There is also an incombustible Stone found about *Miletum* [z], which is of an angular

---

[y] It was from this Property of resembling a burning Coal when held against the Sun, that this Stone obtain'd the Names *Carbunculus* and ἄνθραξ, which afterwards being misunderstood, there grew an Opinion of its having the Qualities of a burning Coal, shining in the dark, and as no Gem ever was, or indeed ever will be found endued with that Quality, it was supposed that the true Carbuncle of the Antients was lost, but long generally believed, that there had some time been such a Stone. The Words of this Author, however, set it very clear, that this Appearance in the Sun only was the Occasion of the Name. That Species of Carbuncle of the Antients which possessed this Quality in the greatest Degree, was the *Garamantine* or *Carthaginian*, and as the Author gives also *Carthage* for the Place whence this he here describes was brought, there is no doubt but the particular Species here meant, is the *Garamantine* Carbuncle of the Antients, which is the true Garnet of the Moderns. Experience shews, that this Stone has more the Appearance of a fire Coal in the Sun than the Ruby or any other of the red Gems, and it is famous for sustaining the Force of Fire unhurt, which is the other great Characteristic of it mentioned by the Author.

[z] The *Miletian* Kind is generally supposed to be that call'd by other Authors the *Alabandine*, as the Places from whence they have their Names are in the same Kingdom. And *Theophrastus*, who describes the *Miletian*, has not mentioned the *Alabandine*, and *Pliny*, who describes that, has not named the *Miletian*.

The other Gems, by the Antients included in the general Name Carbuncle, are distinguished by later Writers into various Species of the Ruby, Garnet, Almandine, and Hyacynth, and are,

ἐν ᾧπερ κ̀ τὰ ἑξάγωνα. καλᾶσι δ' ἄνθρακα κὴ τᾶ-
τον· ὃ κ̀ θαυμαςὸν ἐςίν. ὅμοιον ρ̀ τρόπον τινὰ κ̀ τὸ
ξ ͣ ἀδάμαντ©.

---

1. The *Rubinus verus*, the True Ruby. This is of a fine blood Colour, and of extreme Hardnefs, and, when large, is by fome call'd a Carbuncle. This is from *Cambaja*, *Calicut*, *Goria*, and the Ifland of *Ceylon*.

2. The Balafs Ruby, *Rubinus Balaffius* or *Pallacius*. This is of a paler red than the former, but tinged with a mixture of blue, its common Shape is oblong and pointed. And either this or the Rock Ruby, as it is call'd, a Species of the Garnet hereafter to be mentioned, is probably the *Carbunculus Amethyſtizontes* of *Pliny*. The Balafs Ruby is principally from the Ifland of *Ceylon*.

3. The *Rubinus Spinelus*, the Spinell Ruby. This is of a clearer red than the Balafs, but is not fo bright nor hard as the true Ruby.

4. The *Rubacus*, the *Rubacelle*. This is red, with a caft of yellow, and is the leaft valuable of all the Clafs.

5. The *Granatus verus*, the true Garnet. This is a very beautiful Gem, and was, as before obferved, the Carbuncle of *Theophraſtus*, and *Carbunculus Garamanticus* of the Antients in general. Its Colour is a deep red, approaching to that of a ripe Mulberry, but held to the Sun, or fet on a light Foil, a true Fire Colour. This is fometimes found as big as an Egg.

6. The *Granatus Sorranus*, the Sorane Garnet. This is of an intenfe red, but with fome mixture of yellowifh, or the Colour of the Hyacynth of the Moderns.

7. That Species of the Garnet called the Rock Ruby, the *Rubinus rupium*, and by the *Italians Rubino de la Rocca*. This is a very hard Gem, and is of a fine red, mixed with a violet Colour.

8. The Almandine, a Stone of a middle Nature, between the Ruby and Garnet. This is the *Alabandicus* of

Shape, and sometimes regularly hexangular, they call this also a Carbuncle from its not being injured by the Fire, but that is strange, for the Diamond [a] might as properly be for that Reason called by the same Name, as it also possesses that Quality.

Pliny, and probably the Milesian Carbuncle of our Author already described.

9. The Amandine. This was the *Trazenius* of the Antients, and was variegated with red and white, but is at present little known.

10. The *Sandystrum* of *Pliny*, a Gem now wholly lost.

11. The Hyacynth of the Antients, truly and properly a violet-coloured Gem, and which, if it be now at all known, is ranked by the Moderns among the Amethysts. The Stones we know by the Name of Hyacynths being Gems of a yellowish red in three or four Degrees, which will be more particularly spoken of hereafter.

[a] The Diamond, unquestionably, comes nearest of all Gems deserving the Character of incombustible, it will bear extreme Degrees of Fire, and that for a long time together, and come out unhurt, but it suffers some Damage, if suddenly brought into the Cold after these severe Trials, and much more by the Burning-glass, which is able to destroy its very Nature, and irrecoverably spoil it. And this has taught us, that no Stone can bear Fire in the extremest Degree unhurt.

The Diamond is the hardest and most resplendent of all Gems, and has ever in all Ages been esteemed much more valuable than all others, its Colour, when pure, as it generally is, is that of perfectly clear Water, but it is sometimes found tinged with metalline Particles, assumed into it at the Time of its original Formation, as the other Gems, and is thence yellowish, redish, or bluish, and sometimes, but very rarely, greenish. As the Diamond thus is sometimes of the Colour of other Gems, but greatly superior in Hardness to them, so the common Crystal, sometimes from the same Accidents, resembles them, and is much softer, and of little Value. Crystals thus tinged are what the Jewellers call Bastard Emeralds, Sapphires, &c.

(48)

λγ´. Οὐ γὰρ ἔσθ᾽ ὥσπερ ἡ λίθησις κὴ τέφρα, δόξειεν ἂν, διὰ τὸ μηδὲν ἔχειν ὑγρόν. ᵇ Ταῦτα γὰρ ἄκαυςα κὴ ἀπύρωʇα, διὰ τὸ ἐξηρῆαʒ τὸ ὑγρόν.

λδ´. Ἐπεὶ κὴ τὸ ὅλον ἡ κίσηρις ἐκ ᶜ καʇακαύσεως δοκεῖ τισι γίνεσθαι πλὴν τ̃ ἐκ τ̃ ἀφρᾶ τ̃ θαλάσσης ζωπυραμψύης· λαμβάνυσι δὴ τὴν πίςιν διὰ τ̃ αἰσθήσεως.

The Diamond is compofed of various Laminæ laid clofe one on another, and Jewellers of Skill will fometimes find the Joinings, and with the Edge of a fine Inftrument fplit a Diamond into two of equal apparent Surfaces.

If the plain Surfaces of the Plates of a Diamond be turned to the Focus of the ftrongeft Burning-glafs, it receives no Hurt, even by that powerful Fire, but if the Edges and Joinings of the Laminæ are turned to it, the Stone feparates at them, is reduced into a number of Scales or thin Flakes, and afterwards melts into a Glafs which has nothing of the native Splendor of the Diamond.

ᵇ The Author here explains upon the Manner in which thefe Stones refift the Action of the Fire, which he declares to be by their containing naturally no Moifture, which he has before declared to be eflential to Fufibility, not by their having already fuffered all the Change they were liable to, from their having been before expofed to that Element, as he gives the very rational Opinion of fome People in his Time, and which we fhall eafily perceive hereafter was alfo his own, that fome Subftances, commonly fuppofed in their native State, had certainly been, and had by that means been divefted of whatever that Element could drive out of them, and brought into a Condition of not fuffering any farther Changes by the fame Means.

XXXIII. The Power thefe Stones have of refifting the Force of Fire, is not from the fame Caufe with that of the Pumices, or of Afhes [b]. They feem not to burn, becaufe they abfolutely and originally contain no Moifture, whereas thofe Subftances do not kindle nor burn in the Fire, becaufe their Humidity has been already extracted.

XXXIV. Some are of opinion, that the [c] Pumices have been entirely made what they are by burning; that Kind excepted which they efteem formed by the Concretion of the Froth of the Sea: This Opinion, as to the Sea kind, they take from the apparent Teftimony of their Senfes.

---

[c] The Author mentioning it but as the Opinion of fome, that the Pumice had already paffed the Fire, and by it been reduced into its prefent State, is a Proof that the general Opinion in his Time was, that it was in its native Condition And this feems to have been an Error of the later as well as the antient Writers of Foffils, who have almoft all given it a Place among the native foffil Stones, as if Nature had formed it as we fee it. Whereas there is all the Evidence that our Senfes can give, that it is no more than a Cinder, the Remainder of fome other foffile Body calcined by a violent Fire either fubterranean unfeen, and perhaps fince extinguifhed, or that of the burning Mountains, on and about all which it is conftantly found, and that in vaft Quantities, and the more violent Explofions of which may have toffed immenfe Quantities of it to Places fo diftant, as to make People forget its coming thence, or into Seas, whofe Tides and Storms may have carried them to other Shores, near which no fuch Repofitories of it are fituated, which might yet more puzzle and miflead People about its Origin The great Quantities of Pumices found in this Manner, far from any Fires by which they might have been formed, floating on the Surface of the Sea, thus thrown on it, or perhaps raifed by the burfting of Vulcanos from its Bottom; and fomething altered

E

λέ Ἔκ τε τ͂ πἐί τὰς ^d Κρατῆρας γινομθρων, καὶ
ἐκ τ͂ ^e Αραβικᾶ λίθυ τ͂ φλογυμθρης, ἢ κỳ κιασηρῦ-

---

from their original Figure and Colour, by being washed and rounded by the Motion of the Waves, gave Rise to an Opinion in some, that they were another Kind, different from those of the burning Mountains, and that they were formed by a Concretion of the Froth of the Sea, and in which, as the Author observes, they had the apparent Testimony of their Senses. Many have erroneously imagined, that by this Kind supposed by some to be formed of the Froth of the Sea, this Author meant the *Alcyonium*, and have fallen foul upon him for ranking that Substance among the Pumices. But no one has done him more Injustice in this point than his Editor *De Laet*, who, tho' in his Edition of this Author he does Honour to *Furlanus*, for having justified him in this point, and observed that this was not his Meaning, yet afterwards, in his own History of Gems, &c. charges him with it, L 2 p. 131. *Theophrastus etiam alcyonium, quod ex maris spuma concrescat, Pumicem vocat.*

^d For these there is, indeed, the apparent and unquestionable Testimony of our Senses, that they owe their present Mode of Existence to the Action of Fire, scarce any fossile Substance being of Strength and Solidity enough to bear the excessive Degree of it in these Places, without being affected and altered in its Form by it, and reduced to a Slag or Cinder of such Kind and Texture as its constituent Parts disposed it most readily to fall into. As to those found floating on the Sea, I before observed how hardly the Author has fared about them in *De Laet*'s Hands, but *Boetius* has yet infinitely more puzzled this Cause in regard to him, and seems even to have misunderstood the Misunderstandings of others concerning him, for he tells us, L. 2. p. 400. speaking of the Pumice in general, Ἀλκυόνιον *a Theophrasto vocari putant, quod e marina spuma coactus sit.* And this is one of the many Instances in which

XXXV As also the other, in regard to those form'd in the [d] Mouths and different Openings of the burning Mountains through which the Flames have made their way; and those made by burning the *Lapis* [e] *Arabicus*, a Stone, which when it has passed the Fire assumes the Form of the Pumice.

---

this good old Writer is so strangely misrepresented, that it is impossible, from the Accounts of others, to make the least Guess at what he has left us, the very Word Ἁλκυόνιον is no where to be found in this whole Book, and what he is generally charged with is, not the calling the Pumice *Alcyonium*, as this Author imagines, but the Ἀλκυόνιον *a Pumice*, and even that Accusation, we see, from a careful Review of his own Words, is wholly groundless and erroneous.

[e] In the other Editions of this Author there is the Word Διαεαρυ, where I have given Ἀραβικὰ, the former is the Name of no Stone in the World, and the latter of one very aptly placed in this Class of Fossils, and which all the Antients have described, but this Author no where else has the Name of. There is therefore no question but that this was the original Reading, and the common Text, Διαεαρυ, no more than an Error which got early into the Copies, and has been ever since (as Errors usually are) carefully and exactly preserved. This is also the Opinion of *De Laet*, who, however careless of this Author in his *Liber de Gemmis*, yet is a thoughtful and good Critick on him in many Places in his Edition of this Treatise.

This *Arabicus*, or, as it is sometimes called, *Arabus Lapis*, is described also by *Dioscorides*, *Pliny*, *Isidorus*, &c. as a white Stone, resembling the purest Ivory, which when burnt became spungy, porous, and friable, in short, assumed the Form of the Pumice, and was used, like it, as a Dentrifice. *Dioscorides*, speaking of it, says, ὀδόντων δὲ σμῆγμα γίνεται καυθεὶς κάλλιστον. and Ὁ δὲ Ἀραβικὸς λεγόμενος λίθος ἔοικεν ἐλέφαντος ἀσπίλῳ. *Pliny*, *Arabicus Lapis Ebori similis dentifriciis accommodatur crematus*. And this was so early as in those Times, and even continues yet to be one principal Use of all the Pumice Kind.

ται. μαρτυρεῖν ϗ καὶ οἱ τόποι δοκοῦσιν ἐν οἷς ἡ γένεσις. καὶ γὰ ἐν τοῖς μάλιςα ϗ ἡ κίσηρις. Τάχα δ' ἡ μ̀ ὕτως, οἱ δ' ἄλλως. ϗ πλείυς τρόποι τῆς γενέσεως ᶠ.

λϛ'. Ἡ γὰ ἐν ᵍ Νισύρῳ καθάπερ ἐξ ʰ ἄμμυ τινὸς

ᶠ That all true genuine Pumices are formed by the Action of Fire, I believe, is an unqueſtionable Certainty, but as the antient as well as modern Naturaliſts have often confuſedly placed among them, and under their Names, other Stones of different Kinds, and abſolutely different Origin, tho' ſomething reſembling them in external Figure, the Author does very judiciouſly here in allotting a different Proceſs of Nature for the Formation of ſuch

ᵍ Theſe Pumices, as they are called, of *N. furos*, ſeem not only an Inſtance of the different Operations of Nature uſed in the Formation of the different Pumices, but of there having been Stones of wholly different Kinds and Origin ranked among them. The Deſcription the Author gives of them, proves them to be no genuine Pumices, but natural and original Nodules, or looſe Maſſes of Matter, and covered with a Cruſt, as moſt of the natural Nodules are, but none of the Pumices ever are ſeen to be, nor, indeed, is it eaſy to be conceived, from their manner of Formation, how they ſhould. Theſe were foſſile Subſtances, therefore, of ſome other Claſs, which, as they in ſome ſuperficial Manner reſembled the Pumice, the indeterminate Manner of writing in thoſe early Times, had given Occaſion to be ranked among them. What they really were is not eaſy, at this diſtance of Time, to determine, but the moſt probable Conjecture is, that they were Pyritæ, ſome of which I have at this Time that bear ſome rude external Reſemblance of the Pumice-kind; and we ſhall preſently ſee this Author deſcribing a Pumice, which he ſays is ſomething like one Species of the *Pyritæ*, called *Molaris*; it may

The Places, indeed, in which Pumices are produced, seem to testify the Manner of their Formation; for they are principally found about the Openings of the burning Mountains. On the whole, some Kinds, perhaps, may be formed by the Action of Fire on Stones of a proper Texture, and others in some other Manner; for there are in Nature many different Ways of Production [f].

XXXVI The Pumices in the Island of [g] *Nisuros* seem an Instance of this, for they appear to have been formed by a slight Coalescence only of an [h] are-

---

give some Light into this Case to observe, that *Strabo*, mentioning this Island, says, *Saxosa est & molaris lapidis copia prædita.* De Laet imagines the Stone described by our Author must have been very different from that of *Strabo*'s, because it was liable to crumble to pieces in the Fingers, but as I have already observed, that the Molaris of the Antients was a Species of the *Pyrites*, and as no Stone is so liable to crumble in pieces as the *Pyrites*, when it has lain some time exposed the Air, and the Salts have shot and got loose, I am so far from being of his Opinion, that I look upon it as a Certainty, that the Nisura Pumice of our Author, and Molaris of *Strabo*, are the very same Substance, and that *Strabo*'s Words are a great Confirmation of my Conjecture, as is also the Size our Author allots the Stone, and its Property of crumbling in pieces, which he also observes was not universal, but only happened to some of them, those, I imagine, which had lain most exposed, and the Salts of which had been let loose by the Humidity of the Air, while the others continued firm and solid, as those in *England* and other Places do, while lodged in the Strata they were originally deposited amongst. And this I take to have been the Occasion of the different degrees of Hardness of this Substance which our Author has described, tho' the Philosophy of his Times had not looked far enough into Nature to see the Cause

[h] The beginning of this Sentence appears to have been

ἔοικε ζυγκεῖας. ζημεῖον ϟ λαμβάνυσιν, ὅτι τ̅ ἀ-
ελσκομϟων ἔνιαι διαθρύπ]ον] ἐν τ̅ χερσὶν ὥσπερ
εἰς ἄμμον, διὰ τὸ μήπω ζωιςᾶναι μηδὲ ζυμ-
πηπεϟαι.

λζ'. Εὑρίσκυσι δ' ἀθρόας κ̅ μικρὰ χειροπλη-
θεῖς ὅσον πολλὰς, ἢ μικρῷ μείζυς, ὅταν ἀπα-
μείρων] τ' ἄνω.

λή. Ἐλαφρὰ δὲ σφόδρα κ̅ [h] ἀμμώδης ἐν Μήλῳ
πᾶσα μ̅, ἐνία δ' αὖ ἐν λίθῳ τινὶ ἑτέρῳ γίνε],
καθάπερ ἐλέχθη πρότερον.

---

always hitherto faultily printed in the Editions which have come to our Knowledge, the Honour of setting it right, by the Emendation according to which I have given it, belongs to *De Laet*, whom it is much more Pleasure to me to name thus with Respect than Censure, though an earnest Desire of doing the Author Justice, and finding his true Meaning, the only End I have in view in my Annotations on him, sometimes obliges me to speak in that manner. What is here κ̅ ἀμμώδης, is in the other Editions ἢ κ̅ ἄμμος; which, as Sand was not the Substance here treated of, could never have been the original Reading

The Island of *Melos*, sometime called also *Mimalis*, has been always known to abound with Pumices, and those of the very finest Kind; which it did also in this Author's Time, as appears by his Description of their being light and sandy, or easily rubbed to Powder, from which last Quality, possessed in some Circumstances in a much greater degree, it was principally, I suppose, that the *Pyritæ* of *Nisyros* obtained the Name of Pumice. As from some like Similitude of Substances did the Stones next mentioned here under the Pumice Name, and said to be produced in other Stones; and which, whatever they were, as it is not easy at this distance of Time, and with the little Light we have from the Writings of the Antients, to ascertain,

naceous Matter: What is esteemed a Proof of this is, that some of the Pumices found there crumble in the handling into a kind of Sand, as if they never had been thoroughly concreted or bound into a Mass.

XXXVII. These are found in Heaps, many of them at least as big as can be grasped in a Man's Hand, and sometimes larger than that, when the superficial Part is taken off

XXXVIII. All the Pumices of the [h] Island of *Melos* are also light and sandy, and some Kinds there are which are produced, as was before observed, in other Stones.

I am perfectly convinced, however, from the Account of their being found in other Stone, and that as we cannot but conclude from the Account, unaltered in its own Texture, were no genuine Pumices.

The Differences afterwards assigned to the different Species of the Pumice, are what may be observed in a greater or lesser degree in the different Kinds we now have brought from *Germany*, the *East Indies*, and the burning Mountains, and the Author appears to have been very well acquainted with them. His assigning a greater Degree of the abstergent Quality to that from the Shores than that from the burning Mountains, and a greater than even in that, to that of the Sea, is probably very just, though not now regarded, as the Sea Salt incorporated in the Mass of those, must add much to this Quality.

The Author having now gone through the History of the Pumices, returns to the Consideration of those Stones he was before describing, and from the History of which he had looked on this as a Digression. The Stones here treated of, are what he has before named among the Gem Kind, as I have already observed in regard to the Sense of the Word σφραγίδιον, some of the Kinds of which he observes differ only in their external Figures and Colours, and others in more peculiar Qualities

λθ'. Διαφορὰς δ' ἔχυσιν πρὸς ἀλλήλας, καὶ χρώματι, καὶ πυκνότητι, C βάρᾳ.

μ'. Χρώματι μ̃ ὅτε μέλαινα, ἐκ τ̃ ῥύακΘ, τ̃ ἐν Σικελίᾳ. πυκνός τε καὶ βαρεῖα, αὐτή τε καὶ μυλώδης γίνε) γάρ τις καὶ τοιαύτη κίσηρις, καὶ βάρΘ ἔχͅ, καὶ πυκνότηͲ, C ἐν τῇ χρήσͳ πολυτιμότερον τ̃ ἑτέρας. σμηκλικὴ ϡ̃ καὶ ἡ ἐκ τ̃ ῥύακΘ μᾶλλον τ̃ κυφῆς καὶ λδυκῆς σμηκλικωͲάτη δ' ἐκ τ̃ θαλάσσης αὐτῆς.

μα'. Καὶ πεὶ μ̃ τ̃ κ. σͻερͶΘ ἐπὶ τοσ̃τον εἰρήσω. πεὶ ϡ̃ τ̃ πυρυ̨͏δίων καὶ τ̃ ἀπυρώτων λίθων, ἀφ' ὧν καὶ εἰς τ̃το ἐξέδημ̨ν, ἐν ἄλλοις θεωρητέον τὰς αἰτίας.

λβ'. Τῶν ϡ̃ λίθων καὶ ἄλλαι κϟ' τὰς ἰδιότηͲας Ͷͅαφοραὶ τυῖχάνυσιν, ἐξ ὧν καὶ τὰ σφραγίδια γλύφυσιν.

μγ'. Αἱ μ̃ τῇ ὄψᾳ μόιον; οἷον τὸ ¹ Σάρδιον, καὶ ἡ

---

¹ The Carnelian is one of the semipellucid Gems, and has its Name *Carneolus*, *Carniolus*, or, as it is sometimes improperly written, *Corniolus*, from its Colour, which, in the different Degrees in different Kinds, resembles Flesh with more or less of the Blood in it, and *Sardus* or *Sarda*, from *Sardinia*, the Place where it was originally found. The different Kinds of this Stone are found in different Places, and our Lapidaries make a great Distinction between the Oriental and Occidental, which differ extremely in Hardness. The Antients divided this, as they did also other Gems, into Male and Female (as will be seen hereafter in this Author) in regard to their deeper or paler Colour, both

XXXIX. The different Sorts also vary from one another in Colour, Compactness, and Gravity.

XL. As to their Colour, there is a black Kind found on the *Sicilian* Shores, which is compact and weighty, and something resembling that kind of the Pyrites called the *Molaris*, for there is a natural Pumice of this Texture, heavy and compact; and this is of more Value and more useful than many of the others, this Kind from the Shores being a better Abstergent than the light white Kind: But the most abstergent of all others, is that from the Sea itself.

XLI. Hitherto has the Pumice been treated of: Hereafter are to be considered the Natures and Causes of the Diversity of the other several Kinds of combustible and incombustible Stones, from the History of which this Digression has been made.

XLII. There are, beside what has been already named, among the Stones which are cut as Gems, other Differences, in regard to their several peculiar Qualities.

XLIII. Some of which are in the external Appearance only. Of this Kind are those of the [1] Carne-

---

which Colours, however, are sometimes found in different Parts of the same Stone. The Jewellers of our time reckon four Species of this Stone, the common or red, the white, the yellow, and the beryll Carnelian, the first of these is again divided into Male and Female, and is much in esteem for Seals, we have it from the *East Indies*, as also from *Bohemia, Silesia, Sardinia*, and many other Places, nor is our own Kingdom without it, though I have never yet found any here perfectly fine. The white is a very beautiful Stone, of a fine Grain, and equal Hardness, with many Kinds of the red, it is not perfectly white, but rather what we call a pearl Colour, white with a slight

k Ἴασπις, κỳ ἡ ¹ Σάπφειρος. αὕτη δ' ἐςὶν ὥσπερ χρυσόπαρος.

***

Admixture of blue. The yellow is a very beautiful Stone, often of a fine flame Colour, and more transparent than either of the former, this is found in the *East Indies* and *Bohemia* only. And the last, or Beryll Carnelian, is properly the Male Oriental Kind, it is of a deeper Colour than any of the others, as also much harder, and more transparent. Some of our Jewellers, knowing of no other Beryll but this, name it simply the Beryll, but it ought never to be so called but with the Addition of its own proper Name Carnelian, the Beryll of the Antients being a Stone of quite another Kind, transparent, and of a bluish green, and evidently the very Gem which we now call the *Aqua marina*.

k The Jasper is another of the semipellucid Stones; it is much of the same Grain and Texture with the Agates, but not so hard, or capable of so elegant a Polish, nor does it approach so near Transparency, its general Colour is green, but it is spotted or clouded with several others, as yellow, blue, brown, red, and white. It is found both in the *East* and *West Indies*, in *Bohemia*, in many Parts of *Germany*, and in *England*. I have a Specimen of it found here, little inferior to the Oriental, and better than any I ever saw from *Germany*. Our Lapidaries distinguish it into the Oriental and Common, and subdivide those Differences according to the Colour of the Spots or Veins. The Oriental is much harder, and capable of a much better Polish than any of the others, it is of a bluish green, and the Veins generally red.

The *European* or common Jaspers are, of all Degrees, of green, and variegated with several Colours, the *English*, in particular, are hard, commonly of a deep green, often not veined or spotted at all, and when they are, it is commonly with red or flesh Colour, sometimes with white, and sometimes with both those Colours.

The Heliotrope, or common Blood-stone, is of this kind also, and very little, if really at all, different from the Oriental Jasper, the Colour is like that of a bluish green,

(59)

lian, the [k] Jasper, and the [l] Sapphire; which last is spotted, as it were, with Gold.

---

and the Variegation red, but in Spots rather than Veins, and of a deeper Colour.

[l] The Sapphire of the Antients, here described, was a Stone very different from the Gem we now know by that Name, and was of the *Cyanus*, or *Lapis Lazuli* Kind; but not, as some have too hastily judged, the *Lapis Lazuli* itself *

We shall find by what this Author says hereafter, that these were evidently two different Stones, and indeed *Pliny*, and the rest of the antient Naturalists, if carefully read, will be found to have clearly distinguished them, and described them to be what they really were, different Species of the same Genus. They were both mixed Masses, both blue, variegated with white, and yellow; but differed in this, that the *Cyanus* had the yellow Matter, in form of Dust, irregularly and confusedly mixed among the other Matter of the Mass; whereas the Sapphire was beautifully spangled with it, in regular, distinct, and separate Spots. These were its greatest Characteristic, and obtained in its constant Epithets of χρυσόπαςος and χρυσοςιγής. *it est* (says *Pliny*, speaking of the *Cyanus*) *et aliquando et aureus pulvis, non qualis in Sapphirinis, Sapphirus enim et aureis punctis collucet*, or, according to *Salmasius, in Sapphiris enim aurum punctis collucet*, and others of the Ancients describing it, have Σάπφειρο, λίθος ἔχων σπιλάδας χρυσᾶ ὡς ἐν στίγμασι. and λιθος ωραιος εχων σπιλαδας χρυσια ως εν στιγμασι

Upon the Whole, what can be collected from a careful Perusal of the Antients on this Subject is, that the Stone they knew by the Name of the Sapphire, was an opake, or at best but imperfectly transparent, Gem, of a fine blue, deeper than that of the *Lapis Lazuli*, and variegated with Veins of a white sparry Substance, and distinct separate Spots of a gold Colour.

* *Quam Gemmam Plinius Sapphirum vocat, Cyanus est seu Lapis Lazuli. Boet* 183

The Sapphirus of *Pliny* is much different from our Sapphire, and his Description answers to the *Lapis Lazuli*. *Woodw Meth Foss* 20

μθ'. Ἡ ᵈ ᵐ Σμάραγδ⊕, ἢ δυνάμεις τινὰς ἔχει.

Ths Sapphire of the Antients was therefore not only not the fame with the Gem we now know by that Name, but had not even the leaft Refemblance to it, I fee no Reafon, however, to conclude from hence, as *Woodward* and fome others have done, that our Sapphire was unknown to them, it was unqueftionably of the Number of their tranfparent Gems, though not diftinguifhed by a particular generical Name. *De Laet* imagines it was one of the many Kinds they reckoned of the Amethyft or Hyacinth, but I think it appears much more probably to have been the Gem they called the *Beryllus Aeroides*, as they did, for the fame Reafon, their blue Jafper Ἴασπις ἀερόσα. *Pliny* defcribes the Beryll in general to be (except in Colour) of the Nature of the Emerald, and fays it was brought from the *Indies*. Their Beryll was what we now call the *Aqua Marina*, a beautiful tranfparent Gem of a bluifh green, and there is abfolutely no Stone which our Sapphire more nearly refembles than this, and to which, if it were not allowed a particular generical Name of its own, it could more properly be referred, nor could there, I think, be otherwife conceived a better Name for it than fuch a one as would exprefs, as this did, a tranfparent Stone of a * fkie blue, and (except in Colour) of the Nature of the Emerald.

Our Sapphire is a very elegant, tranfparent Gem, in moft Species of a beautiful blue, and nearly approaching to the Ruby in Hardnefs. It owes its Colour to Particles of Copper diffolved in fome Menftruum of an alkaline Nature, and, as more or lefs of this cupreous Matter has entered its original Compofition, is of a deeper or paler blue, and in the entire Abfence of it, perfectly colourlefs, and refembling a Diamond.

We have now among the Jewellers, four Species of this Gem, 1. The blue Oriental Sapphire. 2. The white Sapphire. 3. The Water Sapphire. 4. The Milk Sapphire.

The firft, or fine blue Oriental Sapphires, are greatly fuperior to the Occidental, and are called, in regard to their deeper or paler Colour, Male and Female. We have

* Sereni enim cœli et lucidiffimi habet colorem. *Boet.*

XLIV. ᵐ The Emerald has also its peculiar Pro-

them from the Island of *Ceylon*, and from *Pegu*, *Bisnagar*, *Conanor*, *Calecut*, and some other Parts of the *East Indies*.

The second is principally from the same Places, and is a true Sapphire, though wholly colourless, being of the same Hardness with the former, and equalling it in Splendor and Transparency

The third is the Occidental Sapphire, these we have principally from *Silesia* and *Bohemia*. They are of different degrees of blue, but never are so well coloured as the Oriental, or nearly so hard, their constituent Matter coming nearer the Texture of common Crystal than the gemmeous Substance of the Sapphire.

The fourth, or Milk Sapphire, is the softest and least valuable of all, this is the *Leuco-Sapphirus* of Authors, it is brought from *Silesia*, *Bohemia*, and some other Places. It is transparent, and its Colour is that of Milk, with a slight tinge of blue

The Oriental Sapphire will lose its Colour in the Fire without any Loss of its Splendor or Transparency, and is sometimes made by this means to counterfeit the Diamond; as the natural white Sapphire is also often made to do; but tho' these are both very beautiful Stones, they want much of the Hardness and Brilliancy of that Gem, and may always be easily discovered by a skilful Eye.

ⁿ The Emerald is a most beautiful Gem, transparent, and of a lively grass green, without the least Admixture of any other Colour, the *Romans* called this the *Neronian* or *Domitianian* Gem, the *Persians* and *Indians* call it *Pachæ*, and the *Arabians*, *Zamarrut*, from whence it is generally supposed the Word *Smaragdus* is derived; though, in my Opinion, there is much more Probability that that Word was from the *Greek* Verb σμαράσσω, *luceo*, or *splendeo*, as this Gem was ever in great Esteem for its particularly vivid Lustre. It has its Colour from some Particles of Copper dissolved in an acid Menstruum, mixed with it at its original Concretion, and will lose it and become colourless in the Fire like the Sapphire.

The Antients distinguished twelve Kinds of the Emerald, some of which seem, however, to have been rather Stones

ἔ τε γὰρ ὕδατος, ὥσπερ εἴπομεν, ἐξομοιοῦται τὴν
χρόαν ἑαυτῇ, μείζω μὲν ὄσα ἐλάττονος, ἡ δὲ μεγίστη, παντός· ἡ δὲ χαριέστη, τοῦ καθ' αὑτὴν μόνον.
καὶ πρὸς τὰ ὄμματα ἀγαθή. διὸ καὶ τὰ σφραγίδια
φοροῦσιν ἐξ αὐτῆς, ὥςε βλέπειν. ἔςι δὲ σπανία καὶ τὸ
μέγεθος οὐ μεγάλη. Πλὴν εἰ πιστεύειν τῆ ἀναγρα-
φαῖς δεῖ ὑπὲρ τῶν βασιλέων τῶν Αἰγυπτίων, φασὶ
γὰρ κομισθῆναί ποτ' ἐν δώροις παρὰ τοῦ Βαβυλωνίων

---

of the Prasius or Jasper kind, as they talk of Emeralds which were not transparent, and of enormous Size, and others no more than coloured Crystals and Spars from Copper Mines, so that a more scientific way of writing would probably have much curtailed the List.

The present great Distinction is into Oriental and Occidental, the former are excessively hard, of a lively Colour, and equally beautiful in all Lights. These are of no determinate Figure, but generally approaching to a round or oval, the largest of them seldom coming up to the Size of a Hazel Nut But these are now become very scarce, and what we have among the Jewellers may much better be distinguished into the *American* and *European*; of these the *American* are greatly superior to the others both in Hardness and Lustre, and are indeed to the *European*, what in most other Gems the Oriental are to the Occidental. They are found in many Parts of *America*, principally in *Peru*. They are often very elegant and beautiful Stones, and sometimes not inferior to the Oriental in Colour. They exceed all other Emeralds in Size, some of them having been found of two Inches diameter. And there are Accounts of much larger.

The *European* are found in *Germany*, *Italy*, *England*, and some other Places. They are the least valuable Kind, and are not only inferior to the others in Hardness, Colour, and Transparency, but also in Size.

perties; for it assimilates Water, as was before observed, to its own Colour: A Stone of a middling Size will do this to a small Quantity only of the Water it is put into, a large one to the Whole; but a bad one to no more than a little of it, which lies just about it. It is also good for the Eyes; for which Reason People carry about them Seals engraved on it, that they may have them to look on. It is, however, a scarce Stone, and but small, unless we are to give Credit to the Commentaries of the *Ægyptian* Kings, in which it is recorded, that there was once sent as a Present from a King of *Babylon* an

---

The true Oriental Emerald is of the same Hardness with the Sapphire, the *American* are very different in this respect, and really of different Kinds, some of them coming very near the Hardness of the Oriental, and others little exceeding that of common Crystal; the *European* in general are of this last Texture also, and, determinately speaking, are rather coloured Crystals than real Emeralds.

The Property of the Emerald, of assimilating Water to its Colour, here commemorated by this Author, has much puzzled those who have written on these Subjects since; they have none of them been able to find it in the Emerald, and that for this plain Reason, that they have all looked for what the Author never meant. They expected to find, that the Emerald would impart a Tincture or lasting Colour to Water, by being infused in it, as vegetable Substances, &c do, whereas *Theophrastus* means no more, than that its Radiations will tinge Water, if made the Medium through which they pass with their own Colour. This had before been observed of it in regard to the Air, and it has been said, * *Inficere circa se repercussum aerem.* Our Author observes, that it will do the same in Water; and, according to its Size and Goodness, diffuse a Greenness through that also, if laid in it.

* Pliny, L 37. c. 8.

(64)

βασιλέως· μῆκος μ̅ τεσσαράπηχυν, πλάτος ἢ τρίπηχυν. ἀνάκειται ἢ κ̣ ἐν τῷ τ̅ Διὸς ὀβελίσκον ἐκ Σμαράγδων τεττάρων, μῆκος μ̅ τετταράκοντα πηχῶν. εὖρος ἢ, τῇ μ̅ τέτρας, τῇ ἢ δύο. Ταῦτα μ̅ ὖν ὅτι κζ' τ̅ ἐκείνων γραφῆναι

με. Τῶν ἢ ᵒ Τανῶν καλυμβῶν ὑπὸ πολλῶν, ἡ ἐν Τύρῳ μεγίστη. ςήλη γὸ ἐςὶν εὐμεγέθης ἐν τῷ

---

[n] There are, beside what is here related, many other Accounts of Emeralds of an enormous Size, though none so astonishingly incredible as this All these I imagine to be either absolutely false, Descriptions of Things which never had Being Or erroneous; Accounts of Things which really have been, but have been misrepresented through Ignorance or otherwise in the relating. Of this last Kind I imagine this *Ægyptian* Account to be, and believe that there really were Stones of these Shapes and Sizes among them, but that they were not Emeralds, but of some other beautiful green Stone of the Jasper or some like Kind.

The Antients, in their Accounts of the Emerald, we find, have distinguished three Kinds of their twelve, as much superior to the others; these were,

1. The *Scythian*, which greatly excelled all the other Kinds, and of which *Pliny* observes, that *quantum Smaragdi a gemmis distant, tantum Scythici a cæteris Smaragdis* The Emerald in general was sometimes, from the particular Excellence of those of this Country, called the *Scythian* Gem, ἡ Σκυθίς by the *Greeks*, and *Scythis* by the *Latins*.

2. The *Bactrian*, which nearly approached to the *Scythian* in Colour and Hardness, but was always small. And

3. The *Ægyptian*, which were dug in the Mountains about *Coptos*, and were sometimes of considerable Size, but of a muddy Colour, and wanted the vivid Lustre of the two former Kinds.

These were the Characters of the three finest Species of

the

Emerald [n] four Cubits in length, and three in breadth. And that there was in their Temple of *Jupiter*, an Obelisk composed of four Emeralds, which was forty Cubits long, and in some Places four, and in others two Cubits wide. These Accounts we have from their Writings.

XLV. But of those which are commonly called the [o] Tani, the largest any where known is in *Tyre*;

---

the Emerald of the Antients, the other nine were, the *Cyprian*, the *Æthiopian*, the *Herminian*, the *Persian*, the *Attic*, the *Median*, the *Carthaginian*, or, according to some of the Critics, *Calchedonian*, for they imagine the Word is mis-spelt *Carchedonii* for *Chalcedonii*, the *Arabian*, called *Cholus*, and the *Laconic*. These were all Emeralds of a lower Class than the three first named, they were in general found in and about Copper Mines, and were, many of them very little deserving the Name of the Emeralds, they differed in their degrees of Colour, Hardness, Lustre, and Transparency, and the *Persian*, in particular, was not pellucid. To these Species of the Emerald, *Pliny* observes, they added the Tanos, a Gem brought from *Persia*, of an unpleasing Green, and foul within. From his Manner of mentioning it not among, but after the Species of the Emerald, and saying that others gave it a Place among them, it is evident that he did not allow it to be a genuine Emerald.

[c] In the old Editions of this Author there was a small Lacuna after τῶν δὲ, at the End of which was αιων, the End of the Word wanting. This Defect had been in some of the first of the more modern Editions, filled up only with the Letter τ, and the Word made Ταιων, but after Editors, dissatisfied with this, and observing that the Author afterwards mentions the *Bactrian* Emeralds, refined upon the former way of filling the Lacuna with a single Letter, and made it Βακτριαιων, in which manner it is now generally received by the Critics, and stands in almost all Editions. I have, however, brought it back to the old Ταιων again, which, from what I have to offer in defence

(66)

ξ Ἡρακλέες ἱερῷ. εἰ μὴ ἄρα ψευδὴς Σμάραγδ(Ο). ἢ γὰ τοιαύτη γίνεται τις φύσις.

μϛ. ᵖ Γίνε) ἢ ἐν τοῖς ἐν Ἐφικλῷ ἢ γνωρίμοις τό-

---

of it, I believe cannot but be owned to have been evidently the original Reading. In this I am sensible I dissent from the generality of Critics, and, as in some other Places, even from *Salmasius*, the best, most diligent, and accurate of them all, and to whom I am much indebted in many parts of this Work; but I had rather dissent from a thousand Critics than from Reason.

That *bactrianus* cannot have been the original Reading here is evident, from the Characteristics of that Species before named, the principal of which was its Smallness. Many of the other Emeralds were at Times found small, but the *Bactrian* always so; its general Character was, that it was too small for engraving Seals on, and therefore only used for ornamenting Vessels and other Utensils of Gold. And it is certain, that if *Theophrastus* had known this Exception to its common Character, he would have named it hereafter, when describing it, and mentioning its constant Smallness. But beside the Improbability of a large Pillar of a Gem usually too small for a Seal, why do those Gentlemen imagine *Theophrastus*, who we shall find hereafter was well acquainted with the Stones of this Class, should suspect the *Bactrian* Emerald to be a bastard kind. It was well known to him to be a genuine Emerald, and was generally esteemed the second in Value, the best in the World except the *Scythian*.

That he could never, therefore, mean the *Bactrian* Emerald here, where he is describing a large, and, as he suspects, bastard Stone, is certain; and that he did mean the Tanus, I think is, from his Account, almost equally clear. He is talking of the excessive Size of Emeralds, and after having mentioned two Accounts, neither of which, he tacitly declares, he can believe, he here adds a third, the Truth of which he seems not to doubt, but suspects the Genuineness of the Stone. *Pliny*, we see, is

for there is there a very large Pillar of this Stone in the Temple of *Hercules*. But perhaps this is no true Emerald, but of the *Pseudo-Smaragdus*, or bastard Kind, for there is such a Stone of that Class

XLVI. " The common bastard Emeralds are

---

just of the same Opinion in regard to the Tanus, ranking it, according to the common Opinion, in the same Chapter with the Emeralds, but not allowing it a Place among them, according to his own Sentiments. That Author has generally copied closely from *Theophrastus* in Things of this kind, and almost every where adopted his Opinions, 'tis highly probable, therefore, that he had read this Passage with Taa, and thence formed his Suspicions of its not deserving a Place among the genuine Emeralds. And to this it may be added, that *Theophrastus*, though very particular in his Accounts of the Emerald, and all its Kinds, has no where else mentioned this.

p After the mention of the Tanus, which the Author suspects to be a bastard Kind of Emerald, and which was brought from remote Places, he now gives the History of the Bastard Emerald in general, which he observes was common, and produced in Places more frequented. What the Ancients knew by the Names of Bastard Gems, were Crystals from Mines, tinged with the Colours of the various Gems, and that by the same means, the Admixture of metalline Particles at the Time of their original Concretion. These had therefore the Colour, and in some degree the Beauty of the coloured Gems, but wanted their vivid Lustre and their Hardness. And thus the Bastard Emeralds here mentioned were many of them no more than common Crystal tinged by Particles of Copper dissolved in an Acid. But though this was the general and more determinate Sense of the Words *Pseudo-Smaragdus*, &c. yet they were often used in a laxer Sense, and applied to Substances of different kinds; more essentially distinct from the GemClass than these, only from their having some Resemblance, perhaps in some Cases in little more than Colour, to the Gems they had the Credit to be named from. And of this Kind,

ποις, διτ]ακῦ μάλιςα, περὶ ᾗ ᾗ Κύπρον ἐν τοῖς χαλκωρυχείοις, κὶ ἐν τῇ νήσῳ τῇ ἐπικειμένῃ Καρχηδὲνι.
κὶ ἰδιωτέρας διερίσκον ἐν ταύτῃ. μεταλλεύεται ρ
ὥσπερ τἄλλα καὶ ἡ φύσις. κὶ ῥᾳδίως ποιοῦσιν ἐν
Κύπρῳ αὐτὴν καθ' αὐτὴν πολλὰς διερίσκονται ᾗ

If I may be indulged in a random Guess, I should imagine this Tanus to have been, which it is evident some had placed among the Emeralds, and of which this Author knew not whether he might not refer it to the Bastard Emerald, though most probably it was no more than a fine Jasper, ranked among these Gems by less intelligent People, from its having a good green Colour, and some degree of Diaphaneity; for I have seen Oriental Jaspers, which, though opake in the Mass, have been tolerably pellucid, and of a beautiful green, when cut into thin Plates.

The Places where these Bastard Emeralds were found, favour very much the general Account I have given of them. The Copper Mines of *Cyprus* could not but abound in Crystals tinged with the Matter of the Mine, and resembling Emeralds. And *Pliny* observes of the *Carthaginian*, that they were always bad, and that the Store of them failed when the Copper Mines there were exhausted. Copper seems, therefore, to have been essential to their Formation, and their want of Lustre and Hardness shews them not to have been truly Gems, but, what I have before called them, coloured Crystals.

Salmasius is of opinion, that Καρχηδ. here is an Error, and that the Word should be Χαλχηδον, and that the Island, the Name of which the Author has not mentioned, was *Demonesus*, in which there were antiently Copper Mines.

Others are for preserving the Word as it stands, and suppose the Island to be *Cothen* or *Coton*, mentioned by *Strabo*, and placed over against *Carthage*. I have every where paid great Deference to that excellent Critic's Opinions, but in this cannot agree with him, because if this be an Error in the Copies of this Author, it is also to be amended in *Aristotle*, *Pliny*, and the rest of the Antients,

produced in Places known and well frequented, especially in two, the Copper Mines of a *Cyprus*, and an Island over against *Carthage*. In this Island the true Emerald is also sometimes found. These are dug out of the Earth as the other, and in *Cyprus* there are many Veins of them together; few, how-

---

who all have it *Carthedonius*, not *Chalcedonius*, and I see no Reason why we should doubt but that there may have been Copper Mines in *Cothon*, though exhausted or lost many Ages since. There are so many Passages in the Antients, where these Alterations are absolutely necessary, that a Commentator who wishes the World to have any Opinion of the Certainty of what they have left us, ought to be very careful how he adds to the Number without apparent Necessity.

These were the Emeralds which in after Times were distinguished into two Kinds, and made two of the twelve Species they reckoned of this Gem, the *Cyprian* and *Carthaginian*, but it is evident from this Author's Account, that they were really no genuine Emeralds, but are two of the Kinds which a more scientific way of writing would have struck off from that List. In his accounting them Emeralds, we see, says they were always bad, and *Theophrastus* tells us, they served as Chrysocolla, for the soldering of Gold, and that some were of an Opinion, which it is easy to see he himself also favours, that they were of the chrysocolla Kind; for he adds, they were evidently of the same Colour. This Opinion was unquestionably very just, and these Emeralds, as they were called, were no other than a larger, clearer, and purer Kind of Chrysocolla, differing from the common Chrysocolla of those Times in nothing but that they were of a brighter Colour and purer Texture, from their having been less of terrestrial or other heterogene Matter, assumed into them at their original Formation. Their answering the Purposes of Chrysocolla in soldering Gold is alone a sufficient Proof of the Truth of this, for had they been real Emeralds, or any thing else truly of the Gem kind, they never could have served for such a Use.

σπανίαι μέγεθ⊕ ἔχεσαι σφραγίδ⊕, ἀλλ' ἐλάτ-
τες αἱ πολλαί. διὸ κ) πρὸς τ κόλλησιν αὐτῇ χρῶνται ξ χρυσίε κολλᾷ γδ ὥπερ ἡ χρυσοκόλλα. κ)
ἔνιοί γε δὴ κ) ὑπολαμβάνεσι τ' αὐτὼ φύσιν ἔιναι.
κ) γδ τ χρόαν παρόμοια τυγχάνεσιν.

μζ'. Ἀλλὰ ἡ μ̃ χρυσοκόλλα δαψιλὴς κ) ἐν τοῖς
χρυσείοις, κ) ἔτι μᾶλλον ἐν τοῖς χαλκωρυκείοις, ὥσπερ
ἐν τοῖς περὶ τὰς τόπες

μή. Ἡ δ Σμάραγδ⊕ σπανία, καθάπερ ἔιρη].
δοκεῖ γδ ἐκ τ' Ἰάσπ ὁ⊕ γίνεσθ. φασὶ γ̃ εὑρεθῆναι

―――――――――――――――――――――

r The preceding Account of the Gems or Emeralds must appear very strange to any one who imagines the Chrysocolla of the Moderns to be the Substance I here class those supposed Gems with. Let it be observed, that the Chrysocolla of the Antients here mentioned, and meant in that Account, was a Substance very different from, and indeed not at all resembling what is at present known by that Name.

Our Borax, which we call Chrysocolla for the same Reason which obtained the original Chrysocolla its Name, its Use in soldering Gold, is a substance which resembles that of the Antients in no one thing but that Property, and is itself made by the Evaporation of an ill tasted and foul Water, of which there are Springs in *Persia*, *Muscovy*, and *Tartary*.

The Chrysocolla of this Author, and of the Antients, was a sparry Matter, of a beautiful green Colour, found in Copper Mines, and in those of other Metals, no where but where there was an Admixture of Copper with the Metal of the Mine it owed its Colour, as the green Crystals and Emeralds do, to that Metal, and was generally found in form of Sand, but when lodged in Masses of other Matter, was always separable by washing or other Means; and when separated, appeared loose and in the same Form. It was in different Places of different degrees of Colour,

ever, are found there big enough for Seals to be engraved on; but the small ones are very numerous, insomuch that they use them for soldering of Gold; which Purpose they serve in the manner of Chryfocolla. Some have imagined them, indeed, to be of the chryfocolla Kind, and in Colour they certainly are very like.

XLVII. The Chryfocolla is found in great Quantity in Gold Mines, and even much more plentifully in those of Copper, and the Places near them.

XLVIII. The true Emerald is, as before observed, a scarce Stone, it seems to be [s] produced from

---

but the deeper colour'd, and such as resembled the Emerald, was the most esteemed. It is described by *Dioscorides* [†] *Pliny* to be *coloris herbæ segetis læte virentis*, and *porraceus*, which is exactly what the Greeks called πρασίος. And *Dioscorides*, in another Place, says the best Chryfocolla was that which was *valde ex πρασιζουσα*, *satiatè porracea*. The Chryfocolla of the Antients was therefore very different from that of the Moderns, and was what, in a purer State, and larger Size, might in those Times very probably be, and really was, accounted a Species of the Emerald.

[s] The Jasper is often the Matrix of the Prasius, and that of the Emerald, this latter is often called the Root or Mother of the Emerald, as that Gem is sometimes found adhering to it. And, indeed, there are often Parts of the Prasius, which, when cut, are not distinguishable from genuine Emeralds. The Jasper itself also often emulates the Colour and Appearance of the Prasius and Emerald. And indeed when we consider what has already been observed, in regard to the original Formation of Gems, we cannot wonder if they are often found degenerating in Appearance, or improving into, and much oftener affixed upon, or in some measure blended into, the Substance of one another. What the particular Stone here mentioned by the Author was, it is not easy to ascertain, perhaps some Stone,

ποτὲ ἐν Κύπρῳ λίθον, ἧς τὸ μ̃ ἥμισυ Σμάραγδος ἦν, τὸ ἥμισυ δ' Ἴασπις· ὡς ὔπω μεταβεβληκυίας ὑπὸ τ͂ ὕδατ۰.

μθ'. Ἔςι δέ τις αὐτῆς ἐργασία πρὸς τὸ λαμπρόν. Ἀρχῆ γὸ ὄσα ὰ λαμπρά.

ν'. Αὕτη τε δὴ πεῖται τῇ δυνάμει, καὶ τὸ λυγ-κύριον. κ̀ γ̀ ἐκ τότε γλύφεται τὰ σφραγίδια.

---

which they improperly reckoned among the Emeralds, perhaps a Prasius, clearer than ordinary, affixed to a Jasper, as it frequently is, as well as to Crystals and other Substances, perhaps no more than a Jasper, finer than ordinary at one End, for it was often found in those Times green and pellucid, *viret & sæpe transluiet Jaspis*, says *Plin, l 38 c 9* and possibly a true genuine Emerald affixed to it, as often to the Prasius, and affixed to, or immersed in others But, whatever it was it is certain, from the present more rational System of the Origin of the Gem Class, that it had been in this mixed State from the Time of its original Concretion, and would assuredly have for ever continued so, there being no Agent in nature of Power to have changed the Jasper Part into the Nature of the other

The medicinal Virtues of the Emerald, according to the Antients, were so many, that, to look over their Accounts of them, one would imagine it deserved even more Esteem as a Medicine than as a Gem They accounted it a certain Remedy, taken internally in Powder, for Poisons, and the Bites of venomous Beasts, for Fluxes of the Belly, the Plague, and pestilential Fevers, Hæmorrhages, and Dysenteries, the Dose was from four to ten Grains. Externally worn as an Amulet, they esteemed it a certain Remedy for Epilepsies, and imagined it had the Power of easing Terrors, and driving away evil Spirits, tied to the Belly or Thigh of Women with-child, they attributed to it the Virtues of the Ægis-stone, of staying or forwarding Delivery, and thought it an infallible Preservative of Chastity,

the Jasper, for it is said there has been found in *Cyprus* a Stone, the one half of which was Emerald and the other Jasper, as not yet changed.

XLIX. There is some Workmanship required to bring the Emerald to its Lustre, for originally it is not so bright.

L. It is, however, excellent in its Virtues, as is also the *Lapis Lyncurius*, which is likewise used

---

to the Violations of which it had that innate Abhorrence, that if but worn on the Finger in a Ring, it flew to pieces on the committing them.

It may not be amiss to have thus once given an Account of the Virtues the Antients attributed to Gems, for they had almost as large a List for every Kind as this. The greatest part of these cannot but be seen at first view to be altogether imaginary, and as to the Virtues of the Gems in general, it is now the reigning Opinion, that they are nearly all so, their greatest Friends allowing them no other than those of the common alkaline Absorbents. However, whether the metalline Particles, to which they owe their Colours, are, in either Quantity or Quality, in Condition to have any Effect in the Body, is a Matter worthy a strict and regular Tryal, and that would at once decide the Question between us and the Antients, and shew whether we have been too rash, or they too superstitious.

There has been more Confusion and Error about the *Lapis Lyncurius* of the Antients, than about any other Substance in the whole fossile Kingdom. What I have to offer in regard to it, is very different from the generally received Opinions, these are, however, first to be examined, for if they are right, this has no Title to be heard.

The first and most generally received is, that it was what we now call the *Belemnites*. This is the Opinion of *Woodward*, &c &c &c how true this is, is to be examin'd from their Accounts, and as they are, most of them, only Copies, and those often erroneous ones, of this Author, he

ἔστι στερεωτάτη, καθάπερ λίθου. ἕλκει γὰρ ὥσπερ
τὸ ἤλεκτρον· οἱ δέ φασιν ὐ μόνον κάρφη κ̔ ξύλον,

---

is, where his Descriptions are long enough, always first to consulted, and most relied on, and from his Words I venture to pronounce it evident, that the *Lapis Lyncurius* was not the *Belemnites*. He first says, it was fit for engraving Seals on, which every one who ever saw a *Belemnites* must pronounce impossible to have been meant of it, its Texture rendering it the most improper Substance imaginable for such Uses. And next, that it was of a very solid Texture, like that of the Stones or Gems, the first Sight of a *Belemnites* must also prove, that this was not meant of it, for it is not of a solid Texture, nor of a Grain, as we call it, any way resembling that of a Stone, but composed of a number of transverse Striæ, and of the Texture, specific Gravity, and Hardness of Talk, which could never give it a Title to what our Author says of the *Lyncurius*, that it was not only hard and solid, but στερεωτάτη, extremely so. Hence, I presume, I may first venture to pronounce this, which is the common Opinion, evidently erroneous, and that the *Lapis Lyncurius* of the Antients was not the *Belemnites*.

The few who dissent from this Opinion, of the Number of whom are *Gesffray, Gesner* *, &c hold, that the *Lapis Lyncurius* of the Antients was no other than Amber. This is the second and only other Opinion worth naming, and the Favourers of it bring many Passages from the Copiers of the Antients, to confirm it. All which serve to prove what I have before observed, that many quote the Antients who have never read them, and shew how useful, and, indeed, absolutely necessary, a correct Edition of this Work of this Author is, in Researches of this kind. This Opinion is even more easily than the other proved erroneous from the Words of this Author, who not only compares the *Lyncurius*, in some of its Properties, to Amber, which,

---

* Ego Lyncurium a succino differre non video: et id quoque pro Gemma habitum olim, præterum quod aureo colore pellucet et splendet, minime dubito.

for engraving Seals on, and is of a very solid Texture, as Stones are, it has also an attractive Power, like that of Amber, and is said to attract not only

---

as I have before observed in a parallel Case in the Note on the Sapphire, is sufficient Proof, that they cannot be the same, as no body would ever think of comparing a Thing to itself. But after having gone through a compleat Description of the *Lyncus*, according to the received, tho' erroneous, Opinion of those Times, of its being produced from the Urine of the Lynx, he begins a separate Account of Amber under its own proper Name, and shews he was well acquainted with its Nature and Properties, and knew it to be a native Fossile. Hence it is therefore also evident, that the *Lapis Lyncurius* was not Amber, and that the generally received Opinions of it are both evidently erroneous. That such as had not read the Antients themselves should fall into Errors of this kind, from the Obscurity and Confusion of those who copied from them, we cannot wonder. But here it may not be amiss to observe, that it is not the Antients themselves, but their Copiers and Quoters of them, who are generally obscure. *Epiphanius*, who was better acquainted with them, has made a different Guess, and is, indeed, the first Author who has had the least Thought of what I shall attempt to prove is evidently the Truth in regard to this Stone.

What it is not, has been sufficiently proved. It remains to enquire, what it really is. The Way to judge of this is, to consider what the Antients have left us about it. What *Theophrastus* says we have before us, that it was of a stony Texture is plain from his Account, and may be confirmed from all those who wrote more determinately, they scarce any of them called it, πέτρα ᾗ or *Epiphanius* has, γεο-... And *Plin.* l. 8. c. 38. ... *candidus, igniculis, glaciatur aesitque* ... *Can any one imagine this a Description of a Belemnites?* All that we find in the Antients about it,

ἀλλὰ κ̀ χαλκὸν ϗ σίδηρον, ἐὰν ᾖ λεπ]ός. ὥσπερ κ̀ Διοκλῆς ἔλεγχυ.

να. Ἔτι ϑ̓ διαφανῆ τε σφόδρα κ̀ πυρρά. Βελτίω ϑ̓ τὰ τ̃ ἀγρείων, ἢ τὰ τ̃ ἡμέρων. καὶ τὰ τ̃ ἀρρένων, ἢ τὰ τ̃ θηλείων. ὡς κ̀ τ̃ τροφῆς διαφερούσης, κ̀ τ̃ πονεῖν, ἢ μὴ πονεῖν. κ̀ τ̃ τ̃ σώματος ὅλως φύσεως, ᾗ τὸ μ̃ ξηρότερον, τὸ ϑ̓ ὑγρότερον.

νβ. Εὑρίσκεσι δ᾽ ἀνορύτ]ον]ες οἱ ἔμπειροι. Κα]ακρύπτ]ε] γὰρ κ̀ ἐπαμᾶται γῆν ὅταν ὀρήσῃ. γίνε] ϑ̓ κ̀ κα]εργασία τις αὐτᾶ πλείων.

---

in fhort, is of this Kind, and determines the *Lapis Lyncurius* to have been a tranfparent Gem, of no determinate Shape, and of a yellowifh red or flame Colour fometimes paler, and fometimes deeper, which diftinguifhed it into Male and Female, as we fhall fee hereafter in this Author; and of a Texture fit for engraving on. Had the Antients meant to have defcribed our Belemnites, they would not only not have named any one of thefe Characters, but would certainly have defcribed its Shape, which is the moft ftriking, obvious, and remarkable thing about it. We are therefore to feek for fome Stone better anfwering this Defcription; and this we find, even to the utmoft Exactnefs, in the Gem which we now call the Hyacinth, which it is alfo evident they have never defcribed under any other Name but this, (for what they called the Hyacinth, was a Stone of a very different Kind, and reckoned by us either among the Garnets or Amethyfts) and which it is not eafy to conceive

Straws and small pieces of Sticks, but even **Copper** and **Iron**, if they are beaten into thin **Pieces**. This *Diocles* affirms.

LI. The *Lapis Lyncurius* is pellucid, and of a *..re* Colour. And those Stones which are produced from the Animal in its native Wildness, are better than those from the tame, as also those from the Male, than those from the Female: As the different Nourishment the Creature eats, and the different Exercise it uses, as well as the Difference of its whole Habit of Body, in being either dryer or moister, make great Differences in the Stones.

LII. They are found, in digging, by People who are skilful; though the Creature, when it has voided its Urine, hides it, and heaps the Earth together about it. The polishing these Stones is also a Work of great Trouble

---

how they could better or more exactly have described, than they have in their Accounts of the *Lyncurius*. I have before observed, that *Theophrastus* mentions more than one Species of it, and we at present know three. *Pliny* seems, in the Passage I have quoted from him, to have meant that beautiful Species of it which we call the *Hyacintha la bella*, a Gem in great Esteem, of a flame Colour with an Admixture of a deep Red, but without any tendency to Blackness. These we have from *Cambaia*, and other Parts of the *East Indies*, and sometimes from *Bohemia*, but not so hard or beautiful as the Oriental. Our second Kind are the saffron-colour'd, these are next in Esteem after the *La Bella*, and are from the same Places. The third are the amber-colour'd, these have no mixture of red, these were the female *Lyncuria* of the Antients, and are the least esteemed of all: They are found in *Silesia*, *Bohemia*, *Spain*, and *Italy*.

(78)

νγ'. Ἐπεὶ ᾗ κ̣ τὸ ʸ ἤλεκ]ρον λίθ@. κ̣ γ̇ ὀρυκ-
τὸν τὸ πὲὶ Λιγυσ=ικήν κ̣ τύτων ἂν ἡ ϛ̃ ἕλκειν δύναμις ἀκολυθείη μάλιϛα δ' ὅτι δῆλ@ κ̣ φανερω-
τάτη τ̃ σίδηρον ʺ ἄγυσα. γίνε]ᾳ ᾗ κ̣ αὐτή σπανία,

ʸ This is much to the Honour of *Theophrastus* I have before had occasion to observe, that in departing from the Opinions of this Author, After-ages became more and more ignorant, their Systems erroneous, and their Accounts full of Confusion and Obscurity, till in some late Ages we have been at the pains of unlearning what our Forefathers had been taught by them, and now have brought ourselves to Systems of real Knowledge, by closer Observations of Nature. In many Cases, we find all that we have been studying for is to know just what we might have learnt from the Works of this Author alone. Of this I have before given some Instances, and the Sentence before us, is another very remarkable one That Amber is a Stone, or native Fossile, the best of the modern Writers seem is certain, as that Gems, Rocks, or Minerals are so It has, however, for many Ages been judged by some, to be a vegetable, and by others an animal, Substance And a thousand idle and incoherent Systems have been received as to its Formation *Dioscorides* thought it an Exsudation of the black Poplar and *Pliny*, of the Pine, and others, the Fat or Semen of Whales And it is but of late, that the World has been again brought into the Opinion, that it is, as this Author esteemed it, a mere native Fossile It is of various Colours, white, brown, and yellow, and is found in Masses of different Shapes and Sizes, on the Shores, in many Parts of the World, particularly in *Prussia*, but where-ever it is found on the Shores, it is also to be found, if carefully sought for, in the neighbouring Cliffs, the Sea having had no Share in bringing it to light, but that it has, in Storms and high Tides, wash'd it out of the Strata of those Cliffs, and cleaned and rounded it at the Edges, by its constant

LIII. ' Amber alſo is a Stone: It is dug out of the Earth in *Liguria*, and has, like the before mentioned, a Power of Attraction: But the greateſt and moſt evident attractive Quality is in that Stone which attracts [w] Iron. But that is a ſcarce Stone,

---

toſſing it about, and rubbing it againſt harder Subſtances. Amber is naturally inveſted with a Cruſt, as the Flints and other natural foſſile Nodules are; it is found in this State, in digging in *Pruſſia*, *Pomerania*, and other Places, and is called Rock Amber. When it has been waſhed out of its native Place by the Sea, and diveſted of this Cruſt, it is called Waſh'd Amber, or Smooth Amber. We have of both theſe Kinds in *England*, the rough is found in digging to conſiderable Depths in Clay, but is commonly of an ill Colour, and impregnated with the vitriolic Salts, with which almoſt all our Clay-pits abound, in ſuch a degree, as often to crumble and fall to pieces, when it has been ſome time expoſed to the Air. The other, or Waſh'd Amber, we have on many of our Shores, particularly the Northern, and that ſometimes not inferior to the fineſt of the *Pruſſian*.

' The Author takes occaſion here, among the Stones endued with an attractive Quality, to mention the Loadſtone, the moſt known and moſt powerful of them all. The antient *Greeks* called this, Ἡρακλια λίθος, and the later, Μαγνῆτις. It has ſince been by ſome improperly called, inſtead of *Heraclea*, *Herculea*, as if it had obtained its Name from *Hercules*, whereas it had it from *Heraclea*, a City of *Lydia*, near which it was found in great abundance. Κέκληται δὲ ἔτι ἀπὸ τῆς Ἡρακλείας τῆς ἐν Λυδίᾳ πόλεως, ſays *Heſychius*. This, therefore, was its original Name among the antient *Greeks*, and indeed its only Name, for the Word *Magnetis*, which was alſo in common Uſe among them, ſignified a quite different Stone. Their Μαγνῆτις λίθος was a white ſilvery-looking Stone, with no Power of Attraction, and in frequent Uſe for turning into Veſſels of many kinds, as the Author obſerves in another Place. And the later *Greeks* calling the Loadſtone by the ſame Name which both had

κ̃ ὀλιγαχȣ. κ̃ αὕτη μ̃ δὴ ζυναριθμείσθω τὴν δύναμιν ὁμοίαν ἔχειν.

νθ'. Ἐξ ὧν ἢ τὰ σφραγίδια ποιεῖται, κ̃ ἄλλα πλείȣς εἰσίν. οἷον ἥθ' ˣ Ὑαλοειδὶς, ἡ κ̃ ἔμφασιν ποιεῖ κ̃ Διάφασιν. κ̃ τὸ Ἀνθράκιον, κ̃ ἡ ʸ ὄμφαξ. ἔτι ᵹ̃ κ̃ ἡ ᶻ ΚρύςαλλΘ̃, κ̃ τὸ Ἀμέθυσον. ἄμφω ᵹ̃ διαφανῆ.

---

from *Magnesia* in *Lydia*, the Place where they were found, have occasioned almost endless Errors in the less cautious Writers since. The Loadstone is a ferruggineous Substance, found in many Parts of the World, and in Masses of different Size. It is commonly found in or about Iron Mines, and among ferrugineous Matter. We have them from most Parts of the World, and there are very good ones found in *England*, there have been many picked up in *Devonshire* and the neighbouring Counties, as well as other Parts of the Kingdom, and I not long since found a Fragment of one, which will take up a small Needle, within two Miles of *London*.

ˣ The Hyaloides has been by different Authors supposed to be the *Asteria*, the *Iris*, the *Lapis Specularis*, and the Diamond, all which seem very random Guesses, and liable to Objections not to be surmounted. The Stone, I think, appears rather to be the *Astrios* of *Pliny*, which he describes to be a fine white or colourless Gem, approaching to the Nature of Crystal, and brought from the *Indies*. His Words are, having been speaking of the *Asteria*, *Similiter candida est, quæ vocatur Astrios, cryſtallo propinquans, in India nascens, & in Pallenes Littoribus. Intus a centro ceu stella lucet fulgore Lunæ Plenæ. Quidam causam non iis reddunt quod Astris opposita fulgorem rapiat, & egerat, optimam in Carimania gigni nullamque minus obnoxiam vitio,* l. 37. c. 9. And Stones of this Kind have of later Years been found near the River of the *Amazons* in *America*, and taken for Diamonds.

The

and found in but few Places: It ought, however, to be ranked with these Stones, as it possesses the same Quality

LIV. There are, beside these, many other Gems used for the engraving Seals on; as the [x] Hyaloides, which reflects the Images of Things, and is pellucid, the Carbuncle, and the [y] Omphax; as also [z] Crystal, and the [a] Amethyst; both which are, in like manner, pellucid.

---

[y] The Omphax was most probably the *Beryllus Oleaginus* of *Pliny*, which, from what little is left us about it, appears to have but little deserved to be ranked among the Beryls, and seems much more properly distinguished by a particular Name, as this Author has allowed it.

[z] Crystal is the most known and most common of all this Class of Stones, our Lapidaries distinguish it into two Kinds, the Sprig Crystal, and Pebble Crystal. The first is found in the perpendicular Fissures of Strata, in Form of an hexangular Column, adhering to the Matter of the Stratum at its Base, and terminating at its other End in a Point. The other is found lodged at random in the stony or earthy Strata, or loose among Gravel, and is of no certain or determinate Shape or Size, but resembles the common Flints or Pebbles in Form.

There are, beside these, regular and hexangular Crystals, found also lodged in the Strata, sometimes pointed at both Ends, sometimes covering the external Surface of small roundish Nodules, and sometimes shot all over the Inside of hollow ones of various Sizes. These last are called the echinated and concave crystalline Balls, and the former the double-pointed Crystal, *Crystallus in acumen utrinque desinens*. The Pebble Crystals of *England* are often of very considerable Hardness, and some have been found there which the Lapidaries have said approached to the white Sapphire. The pointed and hexangular are what Authors have called *Iris*'s and *Pseudo-adamantes*. The Antients were of opinion, that Crystal was only Water congealed in long tract

νέ. Εὑρίσκον]) ἢ κ) αὗται, ᾧ τὸ Σάρδιον, δια-
κοπ]ομβ῀ων τινῶν πε]ρῶν.

νς΄. Καὶ ἄλλαι δ', ὡς προείρη]), πρότερον δια-
φόρας ἔχεσαι, κ) ζυώνυμοι πρὸς ἀλλήλας Τε
γὸ Σαρδὶε, τὸ μ̃ διαφανὲς, ἐρυθρότερον), καλεῖται
b θῆλυ· τὸ) διαφανὲς μ̃, μελάν]ερον), ᾧ ἄρσεν.
κ) τὰ λυ[κε'ρια δ' ὡσαύτως. ὧν τὸ θῆλυ διαφα-
νέςερον, καὶ ξανθότερον. καλεῖται) ᾧ ᶜκυανὸς, ὁ
μ̃ ἄρρ]ω, ὁ) θῆλυς. μελάν]ερ۞) ὁ ἄρρ]ω.

---

of Time, into an Ice, more durable than the common And *Pliny* thought it was no where to be found but in exceſſively cold Regions, but we are now very certain, that it is found even in the hotteſt.

ᵃ The Amethyſt of the Antients was the ſame with the Gem known yet by that Name. It is a very elegant Stone, of a purple or violet Colour, in different degrees of Deepneſs. It is found both in the Fiſſures, and lodged among the Matter of the Strata, and ſometimes, like common Cryſtal, in concave Balls, reſembling the Ætitæ. It owes its Colour to Iron. And common Cryſtal and Spar are often found in and about Mines of that Metal, tinged in different degrees to a Reſemblance of it. The Antients reckoned five Species of the Amethyſt, differing in degrees of Colour, and we have at leaſt as many among the Jewellers at preſent, though they are not at the pains to diſtinguiſh them by particular Names, they divide them in general into Oriental and Occidental, the former are very ſcarce, but of great Hardneſs, Luſtre, and Beauty; the latter are from many Places, particularly *Saxony*, *Germany*, and *Bohemia*. They are often as finely coloured as the Oriental, but are ſoft as Cryſtal. In *England* we alſo ſometimes find them very beautiful, and of tolerable Hardneſs.

The Amethyſt loſes its Colour in the Fire, like the Sap-

LV. These, as also the Carnelian, are sometimes found in the dividing other Stones.

LVI. Other Differences there also are, as was before observed, in Gems of the same Name: As in Carnelians, that Species which is pellucid and of a brighter red, is called the [b] Female; and that which is pellucid and of a deeper red, with some tendency to Blackness, the Male. The *Lapis Lyncurius* is distinguished in like manner, the Female of which is more transparent, and of a paler yellow; and the [c] *Lapis Cyanus* is in the same manner divided into Male and Female, the Male is in this also of the deeper Colour.

---

phire and Emerald. The Oriental kind, divested of its Colour by this means, comes out with the true Lustre and Water of the Diamond, and is so nice a Counterfeit of it, that even a very expert Jeweller may be deceived by it.

[b] The Division of the Gems into Male and Female, from their deeper or paler Colour, I have before observed, is in a manner general, and runs through almost the whole Class, the Male is always the deeper, the Female the paler, tho' both Kinds, as they are called, are often found in the same Stone. This Difference in the degree of Colour happens from the different Quantity of the metalline Particles, to which they wholly owe their Colours, mixed with them at their original Formation. And I make no doubt, but that there are some of all the Kinds perfectly colourless, if we were enough acquainted with their exact Texture and degree of Hardness to be able to distinguish them by it, and that if we were, we should as surely find white Emeralds, and white Amethysts, as white Sapphires, there being scarce any of the coloured Gems of which we do not see the Male and Female, as they are called, and of which some Specimens of the Female are not found nearly as colourless as Crystal.

[c] The Carnelian and *Lapis Lyncurius* have been spoken of already. The Gem which the Antients called *Cyanus*, is

(84)

νζ'. Τὸ δ' ᵈ ὀνύχιον, μικτὴ λευκῷ κ̀ φαιῷ παρ' ἄλληλα. τὸ δ' ἀμέθυσον οἰνωπὸν τῇ χρόα.

---

what we now know by the Name of *Lapis Lazuli*, a Stone common among us in the Tops of Snuff-boxes and other Toys, and of which the glorious blue Colour called Ultramarine by the Painters is made. This has also been already treated of occasionally in the Notes on the Sapphire. To what is there said of it, it may be not improper to add, that it is a true Copper Ore, generally yielding about $\frac{1}{4}$ of that Metal, and commonly a little Silver. It is of two Kinds, the Oriental and *German*, the former is from *Asia*, *Africa*, and the *East Indies*, the Colour produced from this is not subject to Injuries, from Time or any other Accidents the *German* is found not only in the Kingdom whose Name it bears, but in *Spain*, *Italy*, and *Saxony* also, in Mines of different Metals, particularly of Copper. The Colour made from this is subject to Injuries from many Accidents, and in time turns green. The Stone, wherever found, is generally of the same Figure and Complexion, excepting, that the Oriental is harder than the other kinds. It is composed always of three Substances, with which there is sometimes mixed a fourth, a kind of Marchasite, of a shining yellow Colour, and flying off in the Calcination with a sulphureous Smell, like that of the common Pyritæ, the other three Substances, of which it is constantly composed, are hard, fine crystalline Spar, saturated with Particles of Copper, and by them stained to a beautiful deep blue. This is what may be called the Basis, and is variegated with a white crystalline Matter, and a yellow Talk of the foliaceous Kind, but the Flakes of it are so small, that the Whole appears in the Form of a Powder.

ᵈ The Onyx is a semi-pellucid Stone, of a fine flinty Texture, taking an excellent Polish, and is strictly of the Flint Class.

I have before observed, in the Note on the Alabaster, that that Stone had, from its similar Use among the Antients, also the Name of this Gem, and that great Errors

LVII. There is also the [d] Onyx, variegated with white and brown placed alternately; and the Amethyst, which resembles Red-wine in Colour.

---

had been occasioned, by later Authors not understanding always which of the two they meant. But this is not all the Confusion there has been in regard to this Stone, for the Antients have, many of them, described it so loosely and indeterminately, that it is scarce possible, from their Writings, to fix any Characteristic, or say determinately what their Onyx was. And we find, in consequence of this, many different Stones described as Onyxes by the Writers since. It is to the Honour of *Theophrastus*, however, to be observed, that he has strictly and exactly determined what this Stone was, and that if the late Writers had consulted him, instead of being led into a thousand Mazes by the less scientific Authors since, they would never have described Carnelians, and a multitude of other more different Stones, under this Name, but have known, that the Onyx was as much a distinct Stone with him, as the Emerald or the Amethyst, and as different from many of those they have described under its Name, as they from one another.

From his Account we are to determine, then, that the Onyx is a Stone of a whitish Ground, variegated with Zones of brown. And such are the true and genuine Onyxes we see at present. What may farther be added to its Description is, that its Ground is often of the Colour of the human Nail, bright and shining, the Zones are laid in perfect Regularity, and do not, according to the Judgment of the nicest Distinguishers of the present Times, exclude it from the Onyx Class, of whatsoever Colour they are, except red, in which case it takes the Name of Sardonyx. The Colour of the Ground, and Regularity of the Zones, are therefore the distinguishing Characteristics of this Stone. And in the last, particularly, it differs from the Agate, which often has the same Colours, but placed in irregular Clouds, Veins, or Spots.

We have our Onyxes both from the *East* and *West Indies*, as also from *Spain*, *Italy*, and *Germany*, and there have been tolerably fine ones found in *England*.

νή. Καλὸς ἢ λίθ۞ ϰ̓ ὁ ᵃ Ἀχάτης, ὁ ἀπὸ ξ̃ Ἀχάτȣ ποταμȣ̃ τȣ̃ ἐν Σικελίᾳ. ϰ̓ πωλεῖται τίμι۞.

νθ́. Ἐν ᵇ Λαμψάκῳ ἢ ποτ᾽ ἐν τοῖς χρυσίοις ἀ-

---

[a] The Agate is another of the semi-pellucid Stones of the Flint Class, it is of the same degree of Hardness with the Onyx, and differs from it, as was before observed, in the irregular and uncertain manner of its Spots, Clouds, and Variegations, being placed. It has commonly a grey horny Ground, its Variegations are of different Colours, and often most beautifully disposed, representing sometimes, very exactly and elegantly, Trees, Shrubs, and Plants, Clouds, Rivers, and Forests, and sometimes Animals. There are Stories of very strange Representations on some of them, and, indeed, the beautiful Images we often now see upon some, may incline one to believe many of the strange Things we hear of them.

The Antients have distinguished Agates into many Species, to each of which they have given a Name, importing its Difference from the common Agate, whether it were in Colour, Figure, or Texture. From their Colours, they called the red *Hæmachates*, the white *Leucachates*, and the plain yellowish, or wax-coloured, *Cerachates*. Those which approached to, or partook of the Nature of other Stones, they distinguished by Names compounded of their own generical Name, and that of the Stone they resembled or partook of. Thus that Species which seemed allied to the Jaspers they called *Jasp-Achates*, and that which partook of the Nature of the Carnelian, *Sard-Achates*, and those which had the Resemblance of Trees and Shrubs on them, they called, for that Reason, *Dendrachates*. These are what our Jewellers at this time call *Mocho*-Stones, but improperly; for they are not the Product of that Kingdom, but are only said to be brought from other Countries, and shipp'd there for the Use of our Merchants.

Others they have named idly from their imaginary Virtues, as that Kind which they supposed had the Power of conquering the Rage of Lions, and other wild Beasts, they

LVIII. The [a] Agate alſo is an elegant Stone; it has its Name from the River *Achate* in *Sicily*; and is ſold at a great Price.

LIX. There was alſo once found in the Gold Mines of [b] *Lampſacus*, an admirably beautiful Gem,

---

called therefore Λεοντοσέρες, which ſome have imperfectly tranſlated *Leonina* only, and ſuppoſe the Stone to have been ſo named, from its being of the Colour of a Lion's Skin. How much they were miſtaken, we may know from this remarkable Deſcription of it in ſo old an Author as *Orpheus*.

Ἀλλ' ἔτος πάντων προφερέςατος, εἴκέ μιν εὕροις
Λᾶο, ἐχοντα δαφοινον ἀμαιμακέτοιο δράκοντος,
Τῳ καί μιν προτέροισι λεοντοςέρην ὀνομῆναι
ϵι δανεν ἡμιθέοισι, καταςικτον σπιλαδεσσι
Πορφυρέοισι λ. οκαις τε, μελαινομεναις χλοεραῖς τε.

Pliny ſeems not to have perfectly underſtood the Hiſtory of this Species; as he is too often alſo in other Places guilty of Errors, in regard to the *Greek* Authors from whom he takes his Accounts of Things. Indeed it ſeems much to be queſtioned, whether the Stone itſelf be not as much the product of Imagination, as the Virtues aſcribed to it: However, as there was ſo evident a Proof as this, of its having obtained its Name from its ſuppoſed Virtues, becauſe it was πάντων προφερέςατος, not its Colour, I could not omit giving it a Place, to aſcertain the original Meaning of a Name ſo much miſunderſtood.

The Agate was firſt diſcovered in the River *Achate*, from which, as our Author obſerves, it had its Name, but has ſince been found to be the Product of almoſt every Nation upon Earth. The fineſt in the World are thoſe of the *Eaſt Indies*. It is found alſo in great plenty in *Italy*, *Spain*, and *Germany*, where there are ſometimes alſo very elegant ones; *England* is not without them. In general, the *Engliſh* are not good; but ſome few of them have been found little inferior to the fineſt of the Oriental.

[b] *Lampſacus* was a City of *Aſia*, near the *Helleſpont*, in

ρέθη θαυμαστὴ λίθ⊕, ἐξ ἧς ἀνενεχθείσης πρὸς Τι-
ραν, σφραγίδιον γλυφερὸν ἀνεπέμφθη Βασιλεῖ, διὰ
τὸ πειτῖον.

ξ´. Καὶ αὗται μ̃ ἅμα τῷ καλῷ καὶ τὸ σπάνιον
ἔχουσιν. αἱ δὴ ἐκ τ̃ Ἑλλάδ⊕, ἀτελέστεραι.

ξά. Οἷον τὸ ἀνθράκιον τὸ ἐξ Ὀρχομενοῦ τ̃ Ἀρκαδίας ᶜ. ἔςι δ᾽ ὅτ⊕ μελάντερ⊕ τοῦ Χίυ. κάτ-
οπΊερα δ᾽ ἐξ αὐτῦ ποιοῦσι. κ̃ ὁ Τροιζήνι⊕ ᵈ, ὅτ⊕
δὴ ποικίλ⊕, τὰ μ̃ Φοινικοῖς, τὰ δὴ λευκοῖς χρώμασι. ποικίλ⊕ δὴ κ̃ ὁ Κορίνθι⊕, τοῖς αὐτοῖς
χρώμασι. πλὴν τὸ λευκότερον κ̃ χλοροειδέστερον. τὸ
δ᾽ ὅλον πολλοὶ τυγχάνουσιν οἱ τοιοῦτοι.

ξϛ´. Ἀλλ᾽ οἱ πειτῖοὶ σπάνιοι, κ̃ ἐξ ὀλίγων τό-
πων ᵉ. οἷον ἔκ τε Καρχηδόνος, κ̃ τ̃ περὶ Μασσαλίαν,

---

the Neighbourhood of which there were Mines worked for Gold, Silver, and Copper. What the Gem was, here mentioned by the Author, there is no determining, but in all probability, from its having a Place so near the Agates, it was a more than ordinarily beautiful Stone of that Kind.

ᶜ The *Arcadian* Carbuncles of the Antients, were of the Garnet kind, but so deep coloured, that they were little esteemed, and those of other Countries, which were of the same kind, but little regarded among them.

ᵈ The *Trœzenian* I have before observed in the Notes on the Anthrax, was what we call the Amandine, a Stone now little known or regarded. And the *Corinthian* seems to have been only a meaner and worse Kind of it. Toward the end of the Description of this Species, after the Word πλὴν, there was a Lacuna, affording room for a Word of about three or four Syllables, it is here filled up from *Salmasius*, whose Motive for giving the Word δ᾽ ὑπότερον was, that *Pliny*, who has copied this Passage from *Theophrastus*,

on which, after it had been sent to *Tyre*, a Seal was engraved, which for its Excellence was presented to the King.

LX. These are very beautiful, and very scarce: But those produced in *Greece*, are of the meanest and worst Kind.

LXI. Such are also the Carbuncles of *Orchomenus* in [c] *Arcadia*, which are darker colour'd than the *Chian*; but are, however, used for making Mirrors; and the *Træzenian* [d], which are variegated with purple and white. The *Corinthian* is also of this Kind; it is variegated with the same Colours, but is whiter and paler. And finally, there are many others of this Sort.

LXII. But the most perfect and valuable Carbuncles are scarce, and had only from a few Places [e],

---

shews, that he had read or understood it so, by giving *pallidiores & candidiores* for it. And it may be observed in general, that there is no better way of judging of the obscurer Passages of the Antients at this time, than by observing how they have understood one another.

[e] The Antients we find made great Distinction between the different Species of the Carbuncle, some of which they set almost no Value on, and others they esteemed at a very high Rate. This Author has very carefully and exactly distinguished and ascertained the Places of the one as well as the other.

The *Carthaginian* or *Garamantine* Carbuncle was, as I have observed in another Place, what we now call the Garnet, &c. This Place was so famous for it, that it was called by many the *Carchedonius Lapis*, Καρχηδόνιος λίθος.

Quo Carchedonios optas ignes lapideos
Nisi ut scintillent? Publ. Syr.

That the *Carthaginian* and *Garamantine* Carbuncle were

(90)

καὶ ἐξ Αἰγύπτȣ, ᷓ ἐκ τ̄ καταδύπων, καὶ Συήνης πρὸς Ἐλεφαντίνῃ πόλει. καὶ ἐκ τ̄ Ψηβὼ καλȣμένης χώρας

ξγ΄. Καὶ ἐν Κύπρῳ ἥ τε Σμάραγδ⟨ος⟩, ἡ καὶ Ἴασπις ʄ, οἷς ἢ εἰς τὰ λιθόκολλα χρῶν[ται], ἐκ τῆς

---

really the same Stone, is ascertained by *Strabo*, ἡ δὲ ὑπὲρ τῶν Γαιτύλων ἐςὶ ἡ τῶν Γαραμαντων γῆ παράλληλος ἐκείνη, ὅθεν οἱ Καρχηδόνιοι κομίζονται λίθοι. And *Epiphanius* adds his Confirmation of this Place being famous for the Carbuncle, γίνεται δὲ ἐν Καρχηδόνι τῆς Λιβύης. *Pliny*, and other of the Antients, confirm also their being found in *Egypt* and *Massilia*, and *Salmasius* has very judiciously rendered the last mentioned Place intelligible, by altering it from Ψηφω, as it always before was written, to Ψηβω, the Name of a Kingdom in the inland part of *Æthiopia*. It is to be observed, however, that the following Ages grew nicer in regard to their Gems, for two of the Kinds we find here placed among the more perfect and valuable, the *Egyptian*, and (according to the just mentioned Emendation of Ψηβὼ) *Æthiopian*, were even before the Days of *Pliny*, ranked among the meaner Kinds, *Archelaus & in Ægypto circa Thebas nasci tradidit fragiles, venosas, morienti Carboni similes.* And, *Satyrus Æthiopicos dicit esse pingues lucemque non emittentes, aut fundentes, sed convoluto igne flagrantes*, lib 37. c. 7.

ʄ The Jasper and the Emerald in general have already been spoken of. The *Bactrian* Emeralds were allowed, as has been before observed, the second place in Value. Our Author's Account of them, and the Place and Manner in which they were found, has been copied by most of the Authors who wrote after him, though all of them have not been careful enough to do him justice, by doing it correctly. It is evident, that *Pliny* rendered his καθαρῆς τῆς ἄυρας, *telluris aperta*, (though it is not exactly so printed in any of the Copies, but, *tunc enim terra, tosa*, or *tellure interarent,*) because *Solinus* and *Isidorus* have it, *tunc enim ditiss'mo se se facillime intueri est*, and *tunc eam tum tellure*

as *Carthage* and *Massilia*, from *Ægypt*, about the Cataracts of the *Nile*, and the Neighbourhood of *Syene*, a City of the *Elephantines*, and from the Country called *Psebos*.

LXIII. In *Cyprus* also are found the Emerald and the Jasper [f]; but what are used for setting in Cups

---

asperta intermicant, which shews that they had read it *till ut aperta* in him, however our later Copies may have deviated from the old ones. But the same *Isidorus* condemns *Pliny* in another part of this Sentence, by transcribing from him his noted Error, of rendering the τα λιθόκολλα of *Theophrastus* by *colliguntur enim in commissuris saxorum*. The Meaning of *Theophrastus* evidently is, that these *Bactrian* Emeralds were used for ornamenting Vessels of Gold, by being fixed in them in various Figures. That this was a common piece of Luxury among the Antients, and that Emeralds and Berylls, the only other green Gem, were mostly employed in it, as making the best Figure in Gold, is to be seen in many Passages of the Antients.

> *Gemmatum Scythicis ut luceat ignibus aurum*
> *Aspice quot digitos exuit iste calyx*   Martial.

> —— *& inæquales Beryllo*
> *Virro tenet Phialas*   Juvenal.

What the Author here means by εἰς τὰ λιθόκολλα, is evidently, that these *Bactrian* Emeralds, tho' very fine, were but small, and therefore principally used to stud and ornament Vessels of Gold. And this *Pliny* has so far misunderstood, that he has translated it, that they were found in the *Commissuræ Saxorum*. And as Errors never fail to be faithfully copied and handed down to Posterity, this has been carefully handed down to us by every Author since, while *Theophrastus*, who never meant any such thing, or imagined there were any such things as Stones to be found in those Deserts, was either forgot, or accused of the Error.

Βακ]εμανῆς εἰσὶ πρὸς τῇ ἐρήμῳ. Συλλέγεσι δ' αὐ-
τὲς ὑπὸ (τὰς) Ἐτησίας, ἱππεῖς ἐξιόντες· τότε γὰρ
ἐμφανεῖς γίνον], κινεμένης τ᾽ ἄμμε, διὰ τὸ μέ-
γεθ۞ τ᾽ πνευμάτων. εἰσὶ ᾗ μικροὶ κ᾽ ὁ μεγάλοι.

ξδ'. Τῶν ορυδαζομένων ᾗ λίθων ἐςὶ κ᾽ ὁ Μαρ-
γαρίτης καλέμψ۞, ὁ διαφανὴς μ̃ τῇ [g] φύσει.
ποιᾶσι δ' ἐξ αὐτῇ τὰς πολυτελεῖς ὅρμες· γίνε]
ᾗ ἐν ὀςρείῳ τινὶ, παραπλησίως τ᾽ πίνναις· Φέρει
δ' ἥ τε Ἰνδικὴ χώρα, καὶ νῆσοι τινὲς τ᾽ ἐν τῇ
Ἐρυθρᾷ.

---

[g] The Pearl was in great esteem among the Antients.
It was among the *Romans* allowed the second Place among
Jewels, and seems ever to have been a particular Favourite
with the Ladies.

Pearls are produced in many kinds of Shell-fish, but the
finest, and what are properly the genuine Pearl, are bred in
the *concha margaritifera plerifque, Berberis antiquis Indis
dicta*. Lift. Hift. Conch. Our Author seems to have been very
well acquainted with the History of the Pearl, and, doubt-
less, means this very Shell by his ὀςρείῳ τιν' Andiofthenis
also confirms its being this very Shell that the fine Oriental
Pearls are found in, ὃν δὲ ἴδιον καλῶσιν ἐκεῖνοι Βέρβερι, ἐξ [7] ἡ
μαργαρῖτις λίθος I have ventured to add an ς to the Word
παραπλησίῳ in the *Greek* Text, because the Sense and original Meaning of the Author seem to have been so. The
Shell which produces the Pearl is not at all like the Pinna,
and some have censured this Author for saying it was,
which he seems never really to have done, but to have
known the History of the Substance he is treating of much
better, and have said, as I have made it by the Addition
of that single Letter, probably lost in some of the Copies,
that the Pearl is produced in the Berberi, and in like manner in the *Pinna marina*, which it also was, and which
the Antients knew it was.

and other Veffels of Gold, they have from *Bactriana*, toward the Defart. They go thither on Horfeback to fearch for them, at the Time of the blowing of the Etefian or annual Eafterly Winds; for they are feen at that Time, as the Sands are violently toffed about by the Winds. What they find there, however, are but fmall.

LXIV. Of the Number of the Pretious Stones is that alfo which is called the g Pearl. It is not of a pellucid Nature, but Bracelets, and other Ornaments of great Value are made of it. It is produced in a kind of Oyfter, and, in like manner, in the *Pinna marina*, and is found in the *Indies*, and on the Shores of certain Iflands in the *Red Sea*.

The Pearl is no more than a morbid Excrefcence from the Shell it is form'd in; it confifts of feveral Laminæ laid clofely round one another, as the Bezoar, the Calculi in human Bladders, and other animal Stones. When fmall, they are called Seed-pearls, and when larger than ordinary, *Uniones*. Our Jewellers diftinguifh them into Oriental and Occidental. They are found in many Places, as well as in different Shells, the fineft in the World are thofe of the *Perfian* Gulph. There are a great number found about *Cape Comorin* and the Ifland of *Ceylon*, but they are greatly inferior to the *Perfian*, and very large ones have been found about *Borneo*, *Sumatra*, and the neighbouring Iflands, but not of the fine Shape and Water of the *Perfian*.

The Occidental have a milky Caft, and want the polifhed Glofs of the Oriental. They are very plentiful in many Parts of *America*; as alfo in *Silefia*, *Bohemia*, and *Scotland*; and we meet with them every Day in our Oyfters and Mufcles here, but feldom of any great Beauty.

Some have been of opinion, that they were bred fingly, one only in a Shell, and that they thence had their Name *Uniones*, but this is an egregious Error, many being very frequently found together, nay, there are Accounts of one Shell producing 120.

ξέ. Τὸ μ̃ ἓν πλεῖτον χεδὸν ἐν αὐταῖς. εἰσὶ ἢ κ̀
ἄλλαι τινές. οἷον ὅ, τε ἐλέφας ὀρυκτὸς [h], ποικίλ@-
μέλανι (καὶ λόνκῷ)· καὶ ἣν καλῦσι Σάπφειρον.
αὕτη γὰρ μέλαινα, ὀκ ἄγαν πόρρω ᾧ κυανῦ τῦ

---

[h] Fossile Ivory and Bones of Animals lodged long before in the Earth, are frequently dug up in all Parts of the World. These Substances have preserved their Texture, Solidity, and Colour, in different degrees, according to the Nature of the Matter they have lain among: Sometimes they are dug up firm, solid, and scarce altered in Colour, sometimes so rotten, as to crumble to pieces in handling; and sometimes stained to various Colours, from the dissolved Particles of metalline or mineral Matter among which they have been lodged.

Of this Kind is the Turquoise, generally esteemed and called a Stone, but, in reality, no other than the Bones and Teeth of Animals, accidentally lodged near Copper Mines, or Places where there is cupreous Matter in the Earth. This, if dissolved by a proper acid Menstruum, makes the Bone a green Turquoise, of which there are some found in *Germany* and elsewhere. And if the cupreous Particles were dissolved in a proper alkaline Menstruum, they convert the Bones or Teeth into the Substance of which they penetrate, into the common blue Turquoise; which Colour it is sometimes found beautifully and equally tinged with all through, and sometimes only in Spots and Lines of a very deep Blue, but which the Assistance of Heat will diffuse through the whole Mass, and make it as beautifully palely, and uniformly blue, as that found naturally so.

The Word μέλαν in this Place has been always translated black; and *Pliny* copies it in that Sense from this Author, for he says, *Theophrastus auctor est & ebur fossile candido & nigro colore inveniri*. If we may be allowed to understand it as I have done, only in the very Sense in which he uses it in the very next Line, and judge that he means by it no more than a deep Blue, as 'tis certain he there does, where he applies it to the Sapphire, for No-body can

(95)

LXV. These are of peculiar Excellence and Value. And there are yet also some others to be mentioned; as the fossile ʰ Ivory, which is variegated with white and a dark Colour; and the ⁱ Sapphire, which is of a dark Dye, and not very different from

---

imagine he intended to call that black, if we receive the Word, I say, in this Sense, and determine that the Author means to say, that fossile Ivory was white variegated with blue, and remember what is just before observed of the Torquoises only spotted and veined with a very deep Blue, as those of *France* all are, and many of many other Places, till brought to the Fire, we shall understand this Passage, the Meaning of which has never yet been guess'd at, in a very clear and very particular Light, and find, that the Substance here described is the genuine rough Turquoise, which our Author has very properly called no other than fossile Ivory, as perhaps all he had seen were of Elephants Teeth, and seems very well acquainted with it in its rough State. Whether the manner of diffusing its Colour by Fire was known at that Time, is more than can now be positively determined. Most probably it was not, and they looked upon the native blue Turquoise, which they called *Callais*, as a different Substance.

That the System of the Torquoises owing their Colour to Copper dissolved in a proper Alcali, is certainly just, I have this to prove, that by a similar Operation I have myself made Turquoises, many of which I have now by me, and which have been acknowledged true Turquoises by our best Lapidaries.

ⁱ The Sapphire has been spoken of at large already; I shall only add here, that the Word μέλαινα in this Place evidently signifies not black, but deep blue, as I have understood it in the former Line. And that this Passage is a strong Confirmation, that the Sapphire and Cyanus are not the same Stone, since he here compares one of them to the other, And, as I have often had Occasion before to observe, we cannot suppose he would compare a Thing to itself.

(96)

ἄρρεν⊙· κ̀ ᵏ Πρασίτης· αὕτη ἢ ἰώδης τῇ χρόα.

ξϛ΄. Πυκνὴ ἢ καὶ ˡ Αἱματίτις. αὕτη δ᾽ αὐχμώδης, ἢ, καθὰ τὔνομα, ὡς αἵματ⊙ ξηρῶ πεπηγότ⊙. ἄλλη ἢ καλυμ{ί}νη Ξανθή, ὐ μ̃ τὴν χρόαν, ἔκλευκ⊙ δ᾽, ὃ μᾶλλον καλῦσι χρῶμα οἱ Δωρεῖς ξανθόν.

ξζ΄. Τὸ ρ̃ ¹¹ Κυράλλιον, (καὶ ρ̃ τȣ̃ θ᾽ ὥσπερ

ᵏ The Prasius is the Stone known by our Jewellers under the Name of the Root of the Emerald, and before mentioned in the Notes on that Gem.

It is a Gem of the lower Class, of an impure green, in which there is commonly some Tinge of yellow. The Antients distinguished it into three Kinds, the one of a plain green, the others variegated with white, and with red, we often see it now coloured from the other Gems or coloured Stones on which it is produced, but make no distinctions from those Accidents.

We have, however, as the Antients had, three Kinds of it distinguished by Colour, though none of them variegated, they are, the deep green, the yellowish green, and the whitish yellow, the last has very little green in it, and more properly belongs to the *Lapis Nephriticus* Class, as but semi-pellucid.

It is found in the *East* and *West Indies*, and in *Germany*, *Silesia*, *Bohemia*, and *England*, but is little valued any where.

Woodward errs in thinking our Jewellers call this the Smaragdo-Prasus, that and the Chrysoprasus are both, indeed, called Species of it, but are much superior to it in Beauty and Value. The Chrysoprasus is a Stone of greater Lustre and Hardness than the Prasius, and is in Colour of an equal Mixture of green and yellow. And the Smaragdo-Prasus, a beautiful Gem, of a grass green, with the slightest Cast imaginable of yellow.

The Distinctions between the Emerald, Prasus, Chrysoprasus, and Smaragdo-Prasus, are, indeed, very nice, but

they

from the Male Cyanus; as also the [k] Prasius, which is of an æruginous Colour.

LXVI. And the [l] Hæmatites, or Blood-stone, which is of a dense, solid Texture, dry, or, according to its Name, seeming as if form'd of concreted Blood: There is also another Kind of it, called *Xanthus*, which is not of the Colour of the former, but of a yellowish White, which Colour the *Dorions* call *Xanthus*.

LXVII To these may be added [h] Coral, for its

---

they are very just. The Antients, we find, were well acquainted with them, and some of our Lapidaries are very clear in them at this Time And as the History of Gems is at best a thing too full of Confusion and Uncertainty, we ought, of all things, to avoid adding to it, by losing more of the old Distinctions

The [l] Hæmatites is an Iron Ore, and a very rich one, perhaps the richest in the World, for there is some of it which contains more than half Iron It is generally of a ferrugineous reddish Colour, very heavy, and in Texture resembling the fibrous Talcs The Antients had five Kinds of it, some of which are now lost. The *Ethiopian*, which was the most esteemed, and probably meant by the first Kind mentioned here, was of the same Kind with ours. The *Xanthus* or *Xuthus*, ξυθος, here mentioned afterwards, was that which was afterwards called *Elatites* It was naturally of this pale, yellowish Colour, but became red, as all ferrugineous Bodies do by burning

Our Hæmatites is sometimes of a plain striated Texture, and sometimes has its Surface rising very beautifully into globular Tubera, or Inequalities, resembling Clusters of large Grapes It is found in *Spain, Italy, Germany, England*, and elsewhere, that of our own Kingdom is very rich in Iron, some of it yielding $\frac{11}{20}$ of that Metal, and running into a malleable Iron on the first Fusion

[h] The Nature and Origin of Coral has been as much contested as any one Point in natural Knowledge; the Moderns can neither agree with the Antients about it, nor

H

λίθ⊙) τῇ χρόᾳ μ̃ ἐρυθρὸν, ϖϱοϛφερὲς ᾖ, ὡς ἂν ῥίζα. φύε) ᾖ ἐν τῇ θαλάτῃ.

---

with one another. And there are at this Time, among the Men of Eminence in these Studies, some who will have it to be of the vegetable, others of the mineral, and others only Nidus's and Cases to some of the animal Kingdom. It were easy to overthrow all that has been advanced, as to its belonging to Animals, or being of the mineral Kingdom, but that there is not Room here for all one could wish to say. As no one, however, has been at more pains to prove it of mineral Origin than our own Dr. *Woodward*, it may not be amiss here, in few Words, to defend *Theophrastus's* φύεται ἐν τῇ θαλάτῃ, against that Gentleman's Hypothesis, and shew, as it evidently is so, that *Theophrastus* was in the right, in determining that it was a Vegetable, and consequently the Doctor mistaken, in imagining it to have been formed in the manner of Fossils. And this I promise myself may be done even from his own Account. It may be proper to premise here, that it was of absolute necessity to the supporting that Gentleman's System of the Solution of Fossils at the Deluge, that this should be proved to be one, because he gives it as a Certainty, that all the fossile Corals have been in a State of Solution, which, had they ever been vegetable Bodies, they could not, according to his own System, have been. If his System be just in this Point, I have Proofs, that, whatever he might conclude from it, it really makes for the antient Opinion, of Coral's being a Vegetable; for whatever may have been the Case in regard to the fossile Corals in the Doctor's Cabinet, I have one which I very lately took up from 25 Feet deep in a Clay-pit in the Neighbourhood of *London*. Which shews evidently, that it never has been in a State of Solution, and must have been therefore according to his own System a vegetable Body; for there are Numbers of small Balani affixed on it, and that not immersed in, or laid on it in irregular and uncertain Postures (as must have been the Case, if they had accidentally been lodged in and on it at the Time of its concreting in the Waters of the Deluge) but fixed in

Substance is like that of Stones: Its Colour is red, and its Shape cylindrical, in some sort resembling a Root. It grows in the Sea

---

the very Manner in which they are found when living and in their natural Posture, which it is impossible they should be, if ever they had been dislodged from it, as they must have been, if ever it had been in a State of Solution. Nor are we to imagine, that the fossile Corals have been in a State of Solution, because they have often very different Matter from the Coralline in their Constitution, nay, sometimes seem almost wholly composed of such. For we frequently find fossile Wood, which, according to that Gentleman's own System, never has been in a State of Solution, saturated in like manner with the Matter of the common Pyrites, and sometimes seeming wholly composed of it. And this very Specimen of Coral of mine, which, it is evident, never has been in a State of Solution, is yet almost wholly converted into an Agate.

To this it may be added, that after all the pains that Gentleman has taken to prove that Corals are Fossils, and formed by mere Apposition of Corpuscles, not by Vegetation, his chemical Analysis of red Coral, has brought him to a necessity of allowing, that there is something of a vegetable Nature in them. And how can he imagine this came there? When I can be informed how something of a vegetable Nature can be produced otherwise than from Seed, I may come over to the Doctor's Opinion, that Corals have been form'd by mere Apposition of Particles wash'd out of the neighbouring Rocks. But till then must believe, that no vegetable Matter can be produced otherwise than by Vegetation, and consequently, as even himself owns, Corals have in them something of a vegetable Nature, that they are Vegetables, and that *Theophrastus* was in the right, when he said they grew in the Sea.

It is matter of great concern to me, that I am obliged in this, and some other parts of this Work, to dissent from the Opinions of the Author above-mentioned, to whom the World owes more real and everlastingly true Discoveries in the History of Fossils, than to any one Man

(100)

ξή Τρόπον δέ τινα ὐ πόρρω τύτυ τῇ φύσῃ ᾗ ὁ
ᵐ Ἰνδαιὸς κάλαμ۞ ἀπολελιθωμῄ۞. Ταῦτα μὲν
ὖν ἄλλης ζκέψεως.

ξθ. Τῶν ϳ λίθων πολλαί τινες αἱ φύσεις, ᾗ τ
μεϳαλλδομῄων ἔνιαι ϳ ἅμα ⁿ χρυσὸν ἔχυσι κα̣
ἄρϳυρον, προφανὲς ϳ μόνον ἄρϳυρον· βαρύτεραι δ'
αὐταὶ πολὺ ᾗ τῇ ῥοπῇ ᾗ τῇ ὀσμῇ.

ό. Καὶ ᵒ Κυανὸς αὐτοφυὴς, ἔχων ἐν ἑαυτῷ

---

beside whoever wrote, and to whom I am myself so much indebted in this very Work. But Truth is to be sought for at the Expence of the Opinions of all the Authors in the World, and as Dr *Woodward* is an Author so much and so deservedly esteemed, where-ever he is in Errors, few would venture to believe him so, unless convinced of it, either by ocular Demonstration, or the apparent Testimony of the general Opinion of the Antients. Where these have made against him, there, and there alone, I have ventured to dissent from him; but cannot but observe, that he has, in this Case of the Corals, been guilty of that Precipitancy of which he so angrily accuses some other excellent Authors, and when he so severely censured in this matter, in which himself was in the wrong, a Gentleman to whom the World is almost as much indebted as to himself in things of this Kind, he should have considered that it might be his own Fate to be afterwards treated in the same manner another Time, and remembred the excellent *Spanish* Proverb, which advises a Man who has a Glass Head never to throw Stones.

ᵐ The petrified *Calamus Indicus* of the Antients, was one of the starry-surfaced fossile Coralloids, and, indeed, was not named without some appearance of Reason. The Specimen I have of it, very prettily and exactly resembles that Body.

ⁿ The Gold and Silver Ores are of so many Kinds, and such various Appearances, that it is an almost endless scene of Variety that may be found in visiting the various Mines,

LXVIII. The [m] petrified *Calamus Indicus* also, is not very different from this. But these are more properly the Subjects of a different sett of Observations

LXIX. Beside these there are also many Kinds of metalline Stones, some of which contain both [n] Gold and Silver, though the Silver alone is visible, and these are very remarkable, both for their Weight and Smell

LXX As also the native Blue, or [o] *Lapis Ar-*

---

or examining the Specimens from them. Gold, *Woodward* observes, is, more or less of it, incorporated with almost all kinds of terrestrial Bodies And Silver I have seen in almost an infinite variety of Forms, that of *Saxony* is incorporated generally with Sulphur and Arsenick, and has from them an external shew of Gold, for which Reason it is called there *Rot-gulden Ertz*, that is, Red-golden-looking Ore. This is very heavy, and when broken is of a very strong Smell.

Beside these, the common Marchasites and Pyritæ many of them hold Gold and Silver in small Quantities, and are of various Colours, and contain sulphureous, arsenical, and other different Matter, enough to give them both Smell and Weight, and sometimes both, to a very great degree.

[o] The κυανός or Cyanus here mentioned, is not the blue Gem before described under that Name, but the blue Colour used by Painters, and since called *Lapis Armenus,* by which Name alone it is now known. The *Greeks* called this and the Gem both by the common Name Κυανός, Cyanus, and had no other Name for this, but generally took care to distinguish which they meant by the Context, as it is here evident by its Epithet αυτοφυης, by way of distinction from the artificial *Cæruleum* used in Paintings; (for the Cyanus Gem, or *Lapis Lazuli,* cannot be supposed to have been so subject to be counterfeited) and its containing their Chrysocolla, which the *Lapis Armenus* always does, that the Paint, and not the Gem, was the Cyanus meant here. The Antients calling these two different Sub-

χρυσοκόλλαν. ἄλλη ὁ λίθος, ὁμοία τὴν χρόαν τοῖς ᵖ ἄνθραξι. βάρος δ' ἔχυσι.

οά Τὸ ὅλον ὁ ἐν τοῖς μετάλλοις πλεῖςαι ᾳ ἰδιώταὶ φύσεις διείσκονὶ τ τοιύτων. ὧν τὰ μέν εἰσι γῆς, καθάπερ ᵠ Ὤχρα, ᵳ Μίλτος. τὰ δ' οἷον ἄμμυ, καθάπερ χρυσοκόλλα, ᵳ κυανός. τὰ ὁ κονίας, οἷον ʳ Σανδαράκη, ᵳ Ἀρῥενικὸν, ᵳ ὅσα ὅμοια τύτοις.

---

stances by the same Name, has, however, been the Occasion of innumerable Confusions and Misunderstanding of their Works, and that not only among the less careful of the Moderns, but even among some of their earliest Copiers. And we are not to wonder if many are at present misled, as it is now generally thought going very far back if we go back to *Pliny*; when we find that even *Pliny*, who has taken the greater part of his History of Fossils from this Author, has in many Places evidently and notoriously misunderstood him. And of this we have an evident Instance in the present Case, for he has confounded the two Substances called by this Name, and said of the Gem Cyanus, what *Theophrastus*, from whom he translated it, says of the Paint, as I shall have Occasion to observe at large, when I come hereafter to the Passage from which *Pliny* translated it.

The Cyanus here meant, therefore, is the *Lapis Armenus*, called by the *Germans*, *Bergblau*, and by the *French*, *Verd azur*. It is a mixt earthy Substance, of a beautiful greenish Blue, and seems composed of arenaceous and ochreous Matter, tinged to that Colour by Particles of Copper. It was first found in *Armenia*, from whence it has its present Name, and used to be brought from thence, but has since been discovered in *Germany*, *Bohemia*, *Saxony*, and many other Places. Our own Kingdom produces it, and that as good as any in the World, but in what Quantity I cannot say. I remember to have seen it in the

menus, which has in it Chrysocolla; and another Stone, in Colour resembling the ᵖ Carbuncle, but much heavier.

LXXI. Upon the whole, there are many and very remarkable, different Kinds of fossile Substances dug in Pits; some of which consist of an argillaceous Matter, as ᑫ *Ochre*, and *Reddle*, others of a sandy, as *Chrysocolla* and the *Lapis Armenus*; and others as it were of Ashes, as ʳ *Sandarach*, *Orpiment*, and others of that Kind

---

Fissures of Stone, among some of the Talcs, not far from *Mountsorrel* in *Leicestershire*, and have of it, which I brought thence.

ᵖ The Stone next mentioned, and said to resemble the Carbuncle, but to be heavier, was probably of the Cinnabar kind, of which hereafter. Some Specimens of this Fossil I have seen of a very fine Texture, and beautiful Colour; and all of it has the other Quality here mentioned, Weight.

ᑫ Ochre and Reddle are Earths of the same Nature and Texture, and only differ in Colour, there are many kinds of each, several of which will be spoken of hereafter. They are all of a fine argillaceous Texture, commonly easily crumbling to pieces, and staining the Fingers in handling. They are used in Medicine and by the Painters. The common yellow Ochre is a cheap and very useful Colour: And the common Reddle is often sold in the Druggists Shops either in its native State, if pale enough, as it sometimes is, or mixed with Whiting, under the Name of Bole Armeniac

The Ochres all contain more or less Iron, for the yellow ones will all become red by burning.

ʳ Sandarach and Orpiment are also two Substances of the same Nature and Texture, differing in Colour, like the Ochre and Reddle, and, in like manner, the yellow will become red by burning.

(104)

οϛ'. Καὶ τ̃ μ̃ τοιύτων πλείυς ἄν τις λάβοι τὰς ἰδιότητας. ἔνιαι ʝ λίθοι κ̀ τὰς τοιαύτας ἔχυσι δυνάμεις, εἰς τὸ μὴ πάχειν, ὥσπερ εἴπομϑμ. οἷον τὸ μὴ γλύφεϑ σιδήροις, ἀλλὰ λίθοις ετέροις ʳ.

ογ'. Ὅλως μ̃, ἡ κ̀ τὰς ἐργασίας κ̀ τ̃ μειζόνων λίθων πολλὴ διαφορά. ἄλλοι περιτοὶ γάρ· οἱ ʝ γλυπτοὶ, καθάπερ ἐλέχθη, κ̀ τορνωτοὶ τυγχάνυσι, καθάπερ κ̀ ἡ ʳ Μαγνῆτις αὐτὴ λίθ⊙, ἡ ϲ

Orpiment is the Ἀρσενικὸν of the antient, and Ἀρσενικὸν of the later Greeks. The *Arabians* call it *Zarnich Asfar*. It is a very beautiful Substance, composed of large Flakes, resembling those of the *Lapis Specularis*, but of a glorious Yellow, very weighty, and sometimes holding a small Quantity of Gold.

There are, beside this fine Orpiment, two other less beautiful Kinds, the one composed of an impurer Substance, resembling common Sulphur, spangled all over with small Flakes of the fine foliaceous Kind, the other more impure than the last, and tinged of a paler or deeper Green in many Places, from Particles of Copper. These are what may be called the three different Kinds of this Fossil; but there are, beside these, almost endless Varieties of it, in regard to its deeper or paler Colour, and the extraneous Matters contained in it.

Yellow Orpiment burns to a Redness in the Fire, emitting a nauseous Smell, and this red Mass is sometimes called red Orpiment. But the genuine and natural red Orpiment is the Sandarach here mentioned, this the *Arabians* call *Zarnich-Ahmer*, it is of the same Nature with the former, but generally in larger Masses, and not of that foliaceous Texture, but in more compact Globes.

All the Kinds of Orpiment and Sandarach are found in

LXXII. Many other Properties there alſo are in theſe Subſtances, which are eaſily obſerved. As that ſome of the Stones before named are of ſo firm a Texture, that they are not ſubject to Injuries, and are not to be cut by Inſtruments of Iron, but only by other Stones ˢ.

LXXIII. On the whole, there is a great Difference in the Texture of the larger Stones; as may be learnt from the different Manners in which they may be worked; ſome may be cut, others engraved on, and ſhaped, as before obſerved, by the Turner's Inſtruments, as the ᵗ Magnet Gem, a Stone

---

the Mines of Gold, Silver, and Copper, and ſometimes two or more of them mixed in the ſame Glebe. I have, from the Mines of *Goſſelaer* in *Saxony*, a moſt elegant piece of the foliaceous Orpiment, which has two fine Veins of native Sandarach running acroſs it. It was brought to me under the Name of a Gold Ore, and I believe really does contain a ſmall Quantity of that Metal.

ˢ This is a Doctrine well known to our Lapidaries, and without the Knowledge of which the Diamond, the firſt and fineſt of all Gems, never could have been worked into Form at all, for nothing will cut it but itſelf. Other Gems and Stones are either work'd with Diamond-powder, or with that of Emery, one of the hardeſt Subſtances in nature except the Diamond, and afterwards with Tripoly, and other ſofter Powders.

ᵗ The Magnet Gem, or Μαγνῆτις λίθος of the antient Greeks, I have before obſerved, was a Stone of an entirely different Nature from the Loadſtone, which we now call the Magnet. The Stone here meant, was a very bright white Subſtance, ſo nearly reſembling Silver in appearance, that it was not, at firſt ſight, to be diſtinguiſhed from it. It was found in large Maſſes, and was of a Texture eaſily to be wrought into any Shape or Figure. This made it in great Eſteem among the Antients, and in conſtant Uſe,

ὄψῃ πειτὸν ἔχεσα· καὶ, ὥς γε δή τινες θαυμάζεσι, τὴν ὁμοίωσιν τῷ ἀργύρῳ μηδαμῶς ἔσαν ζυγγενῆ.

οδ΄. Πλείες δ' εἰσὶν οἱ δεχόμενοι πάσας τὰς ἐργασίας. ἐπεὶ κ̀ ἐν Σίφνῳ πιετός τις ἐσὶν ὀρυκτές. ὡς -ρία σάδια ἀπὸ θαλάτης, ςρογγύλ@. κ̀ βωλώδης. κ̀ τορνεύεται, καὶ γλύφε) διὰ τὸ μαλακὸν. ὅταν ὀ πυρωθῇ (κὰ ἀποβαφῇ) τῷ ἐλαίῳ, μέλας τε σφόδρα γίνε), κ̀ ζηρός. ποιεσι δ' ἐξ αὐτε κυλίη τὰ ἐπιτράπεζα.

Οἱ μ πιετοὶ πάντες ὑποδέχον) τὴν ε σιδήρε δύναμιν. ἔνιοι ὀ λίθοις ἄλλοις γλύφον), σίδηρ@ δ' ε δύνα). καθάπερ εἴπομεν. οἱ ὀ σιδήροις μ ἀμβλέσι ὀ καί εἰσιν, ὥςτε παραπλησίως ὀ κ̀ τὸ μὴ τέμνεσθ σιδήρῳ.

---

turned into Veſſels of different kinds. What Stone it was, is at preſent not to be certainly determined, probably it may be now loſt, at leaſt among the Nations we have commerce with.

What I have before obſerved of the Antients calling this ſilvery Stone the Magnet, and our Loadſtone the *Heraclius Lapis*, is confirmed, in very plain Words, by *Heſychius*, Μαγνῆτις λίθος, αὕτη παλαιᾶ τιν ὄψιν ἀργυρῳ ἐμφερὴς ἔσα, ἡ δὲ Ἡρακλεῶτις τὸν σίδηρον ἐπισπᾶται

This Stone was afterwards called *Lapis Siphrius*, from the Place where our Author obſerves it was found, which was an Iſland in the *Ægean Sea*, called by ſome *Merope*. What the Antients in general have left us about it beſide,

of very elegant Appearance, and much admired by many: This carries a fine Resemblance of Silver, though it is in reality a Stone of an entirely different Kind.

LXXIV. Many also there are, which admit all Kinds of working, as in [v] *Siphnus* there is a fossile Substance of this kind, which is dug in Lumps, and roundish Masses, at about three Furlongs distance from the Sea: This may at first be either engraved on, or worked by the Turner into any Form by reason of its Softness; but when it is afterwards burnt and wetted with Oil, it becomes black and solid. Vessels of different kinds, for the service of the Table, are made of this.

LXXV. All Substances of this kind are to be worked on by Iron Instruments, but others there are, which, as before observed, will not be touch'd by them, but must be cut by other Stones, and others yet, which may be cut with Iron, but the Instruments must be dull and blunt[w]. Which is much as if they were not cut by Iron.

---

is, that it was of strength to bear the Fire. And Vessels made of it, served, as those of Earthen-ware, for the common Offices of Boiling, &c. *Pliny* sums up their Accounts of it in these Words *In Siphno Lapis est qui cavatur, tornaturque in vasa coquendis cibis utilia, vel ad esculentorum usus*, and a little afterwards, *Sed in Siphnio singulare quod, excalfactus, oleo nigrescit durescitque, natura mollissimus.*

[w] The Marbles, Alabasters, and most other Stone of Strata, are of the Number of those which we cut with blunt Iron Instruments. But if we consider our Manner of performing this, which probably is the same that was used in this Author's Time, and is not without the As-

οε. Καί τοι ὴ ϛερεώτερα ὴ ἰχυρότερα τέμνᾳ ὴ σίδηρ۞, λίθυ ϛκληρότερ۞ ὤν.

οζ. Ἄτοπον ϑ̓ κἀκείνῳ φαίνε]· διότι ἡ μ̃ ἀκόνη κα]εϛϑίει τ̃ σίδηρον, ὁ ϑ̓ σιδηρ۞ ταύτην μ̃ δύνα-ται διαίρειν ὴ ῥυθμίζειν, ἐξ ἧς δ̓ αἱ σφραγίδες, ὔ. ὴ πάλιν, ὁ λίθ۞, ᾧ γλύφυσι τὰς σφραγίδας, ἐκ τύτυ ἐϛὶν ἐξ ὅπερ αἱ ἀκόναι, ἢ ἐξ ὁμοία τύ-τῳ. ἄγε] δ̓ ἡ ἐξ Ἀρμϑνίας ˣ.

---

fiſtance of Water and Sand, we ſhall find, that theſe are not properly to be divided from the Claſs of thoſe uſually cut with other Stones, for, in reality, the Sand in this Caſe does more than the Iron, and is a ſimilar Subſtance to the Powder of hard Stones uſed to Gems, tho' coarſer. The Art of cutting and poliſhing the harder Gems with other Stones was known very early in the World. We have Accounts from ſome of the earlieſt Authors, of Fragments of Diamonds being ſet in a convenient manner for hand-ling, and made into Tools for the working on other Gems with. Diamond-powder is the great thing in uſe with us on theſe Occaſions, and next to it Emery, and Emery was alſo known to the Antients, and uſed by them on the ſame Occaſions. Σμίρις λίθος ἐϛὶν ἤ τὰς ψήφυς οἱ δακτυλιογλύφοι σμή-χυσι, Dioſcorides. Σμίρις ἀμμυ εἶδος, ἤ σμηχο]αι σκληροὶ τῶν λί-θων, Heſychius.

Cardanus imagines, but erroneouſly, that the Porus of the Antients was our Emery, or elſe, that our Emery was unknown to them, which is no leſs an Error. For it is evident, they were well acquainted with its Uſes. And what he adds, of their working on Gems with the Porus, and Fragments of the Lapis Obſidianus, Salmaſius, who had certainly read more than moſt Men, affirms, he never

LXXVI. Iron, however, being harder in its Texture than Stone, will cut such as are both harder and more solid than these.

LXXVII. There seems, however, yet an Absurdity in this, since the Whetstone has Power upon, and takes off a Part of the Iron Instruments which are sharpened on it, and the Instrument may be made to cut and work upon the Whetstone; but notwithstanding, will not cut those Gems which are work'd into Seals, tho' the Stone with which they are worked is composed of the same kind of Matter with the Whetstone, or something not very unlike it. These Stones are from *Armenia* [x].

---

could find any Account of among them. *Pliny* relates, indeed, that Fragments of the harder kind of the *Ostracites* were used for this Purpose, lib. 37. c. 10. *Ostracia seu Ostracites est testacea durior alteraa Achatæ similis nisi quòd Achates politura pinguescit; durior tanta inest vis ut aliæ omnia scalpantur fragmentis ejus.* And that a Sand prepared from the Porus, was used for polishing Marble, but not Gems, *Cissior enim harena laxioribus segmentis terit, & plus erodit marmoris, majusque opus scabritiæ politurae relinquit. Rursus Theleica polituris accommodatur, & quae fit e poro lapide aut e pumice.* For *poro lapide*, many of the Copies have *toro lapide*, and *duro lapide*, but the concurrent Accounts of other of the Antients determine it to be this particular Stone that is meant. And the same Author expresly says, that the *Obsidianus* could not cut the true Gems, *Obsidianae fragmenta veras gemmas non scarifant*.

[x] The *Armenian* Whetstones, *Coticulæ* of the *Latins*, and ἀγίαι of the *Greeks*, were of a Stone of extreme Hardness, and, as we may learn from this Passage, of the same Nature with that, which they used for the working some of those Stones which Iron could not touch.

This Stone used for working on others they first had from *Cyprus*, and some of the antient *Greeks* called it *A-*

σή. Θαυμαςὴ ἡ φύσις καὶ τῆ βασανιζάσης τὸν
ʸ χρυσόν. δοκεῖ γὰ ἡ τὴν τοιαύτην ἔχειν τῷ πυρὶ
δύναμιν, ᾗ γὰ ἐκεῖνο δοκιμάζει. διὸ καὶ ἀπορῶσί τι-

---

damas, from its extreme Hardness, as they also did sometimes Iron for the same Reason. Which Manner of writing has much misled their Copiers, and even *Pliny*, who, after having in one Place given the right Account of this Stone, and called it *Cos*, in another mistakes it for a Diamond, and calls it such. This was the Effect of his copying from different Authors in different parts of his Work, and not seeing in many Places that they were describing only the same Substance under two different Names. This *Cyprian* Stone was long in esteem, and served not only for polishing, but boring Holes through such Gems as they strung on Threads, to wear as Bracelets, and other the like Ornaments. But After-ages found out the *Armenian*, which proving much harder than it, became more generally used, and at length entirely banished the other. That this *Armenian* was of the same Kind with their Ἀκόναι, is evident from this Passage of *Theophrastus*, and that it had the Properties of the *Cyprian*, and was used as it, is plain from *Stephanus*'s Account of it, παρέχολαι δὲ λίθον τὴν γλύφυσαι κʲ τρυπῶσαι τὰς σφραγῖδας. *Pliny*'s Account of other Gems being bored by *Cyprian* Diamonds, means no more, than that they were worked by a Stone of the Nature of the Ἀκόνη, brought from *Cyprus*.

ʸ The Stone here described is the *Lapis Lydius* of Author, commonly called the Touch-stone, from its Office of trying Metals by the Touch. The excellent *Salmasius*, generally so happy in understanding the Antients, and to whom I am obliged, in the course of this Work, much oftner than to any other Author, is guilty of a Mistake in regard to this Stone, and erroneously accuses *Pliny* of a great Error, in a thing in which that Author, however often faulty, is perfectly right. Errors in the Works of Men of such Eminence as this excellent Critic, ought above all things, to be set right, as they otherwise pass with the generality of Readers as certain and unquestionable Truths. And

LXXVIII. The Nature of the Stone which tries y Gold is also very wonderful, as it seems to have the same Power with Fire; which is also a Test of that Metal Some People have, for this Reason,

---

this, in particular, being in the Name of a Stone, ought to be cleared rather than any other, as Errors about Names are what alone have given more than half the Confusion we have, in regard to the Works of the Antients Pliny has said of this Stone, *Auri argentique mentionem comitatur lapis, quem coticulam appellant, quondam non solitus inveniri nisi in flumine Tmolo, ut auctor est Theophrastus nunc vero passim, quem alii Heraclium, alii Lydium vocant.* On which Salmasius's Remark is this, *Fallitur Plinius peccatque non mediocriter. Lapis hic Lydius quo aurum & argentum probatur, nunquam dictus est Heraclius, sed ille alter Lydius qui ferrum rapit* I am sorry to say it, but it is *fallitur Salmasius*, not *Plinius*, for we need look no farther than this Author to know, that *Heraclius* was as common a Name for the Touchstone among the Antients, as for the Loadstone, see *p* 16, where he expressly says, that the Touchstone was so called, οἱ δὲ βασανίζειν τὸν ἄργυρον ὥσπερ ἤτε καλεῖ ἡ λίθος Ἡρακλεία καὶ ἡ Λυδή The Loadstone and Touchstone were therefore both called, among the Antients, from their common Country, *Lapis Lydius*, and *Lapis Heraclius* And for that Reason there have been great Errors in regard to them, in many of the less careful Writers since. As about the two Cyanus's, and, in short, all the Substances which they had thus confused, in not allowing particular Names to. It has since been called *Lapis Basanites*, from its Use in trying Metals, *Chrysites*, from its particular Efficacy in tryal of Gold, and *Cotula*, because it was generally formed, for Conveniency, into the Shape of a small Whetstone We are not to suppose, however, that this Stone alone serves for this Purpose, in *Italy* a green Marble, called there *Verdello*, is now generally used in its stead, and in most other Places the *Basaltes*, a black M , found in regularly shaped Columns, many placed together, as in *Ireland*, where a Quantity of it is called the Giants Causeway.

νες, ὀκ ἄγαν οἰκείως ἀπορῦντες. ὐ ʝὸ τ' αὐτὸν τρόπον δοκιμάζει. ἀλλα τὸ μ῀ πῦρ τῷ τὰ χρώματα μεταβάλλειν, κ᾽ ἀξιῦν. ὁ ὃ λίθ@, τῇ παρατρίψ͵. δύνας γὰρ, ὡς ἔοικεν, ἐκλαμβάνειν τὴν ἑκάςυ φύσιν

οθ'. Εὑρῆας δέ φασιν νῦν ἀμείνω πολὺ τ῀ πρότερον. ὥςε μὴ μόνον τ῀ ἐκ τ῀ καθάρσεως, ἀλλὰ κ᾽ τ῀ χαλκὸν καὶ ἄχρυσον, ἀργυρον γνωρίζειν, κ᾽ πόσον εἰς τ῀ ςατῆρα μέμικ]. σημεῖα δ' ἐςὶν αὐτοῖς ἀπὸ ϟ ἐλαχίςυ. ἐλάχιςον ὃ γίνε] κερβὴ, εἶτα κόλυβον. εἶτα τεταρτημόριον, ἢ ἡμιόβολ@. ἐξ ὧν γνωρίζυσι τὸ καθῆκον.

π'. Εὑρίσκον] ᾽ τιαῦται πᾶσαι ἐν τῷ ποταμῷ [z] Τμολῷ λεία δ᾽ ἡ φύσις αὐτῶν καὶ ψηφοειδὴς, πλατεῖα, ὐ ςρογγύλη. μέγεθ@ δέ ἐςιν διπλασία τ῀ μεγίςης ψήφυ. Διαφέρᾳ δ᾽ αὐτῆς πρὸς τὴν δοκιμασίαν τὰ ἄνω πρὸς τ᾽ ἥλιον, ἢ τὰ κάτω. κ᾽ βέλτιον δοκιμάζει τὰ ἄνω. τῦτο δέον, ὅτι ξηρότερα

---

[z] The true *Lydius* was originally found only in this River, afterwards in many other Places, and at present is very plentiful in many of the larger Rivers of *Germany*. This Author gives a very circumstantial Account of the
Pro-

questioned the Truth of this Power in the Stone; but their Doubts are ill founded, for this Tryal is not of the same Nature, or made in the same Manner with the other. The Tryal by Fire is by the Colour, and Quantity lost by it; but that by the Stone, is made only by rubbing the Metal on it; the Stone seeming to have a Power of receiving separately the distinct Particles of different Metals.

LXXIX. It is said also, that there is a much better kind of this Stone now found out, than that which was formerly used, insomuch, that it now serves not only for the Tryal of the refined Gold, but also of Copper or Silver coloured with Gold; and shews how much of the adulterating Matter by weight is mixed with Gold. This has Signs which it yields from the smallest Weight of the adulterating Matter, which is a Grain, from thence a Colybus, and thence a Quadrans or Semi-Obolus; by which it is easy to distinguish if, and in what degree, that Metal is adulterated.

LXXX. All these Stones are found in the River *Tmolus*, their Texture is smooth, and like that of Pebbles, their Figure broad not round, and their Bigness twice that of the common larger sort of Pebbles. In their Use in the Tryal of Metals, there is a Difference in Power between their upper Surface, which has lain toward the Sun, and their under, which has been to the Earth, the upper performing its Office the more nicely, and this is

---

Property of this Stone, and they had in his Time very good ones, and knew very well how to use them, if they could do what he says with them.

τὰ ἄνω. κωλύει γὰρ ἡ ὑγρότης εἰς τὸ ἐκλαμβάνειν. ἐπειδὴ κ̓ ἐν τοῖς καύμασι τὸ δοκιμάζειν χεῖρον. ἀνίησι γάρ τινα νοτίδα ἐξ αὑτῆς. δι᾽ ἣν ἀπολιθαίνῃ. ζυμβαίνει ϑ̓ τῦτο κ̓ ἄλλοις τ῀ λίθων. ἐξ ὧν τὰ ἀγάλματα ποιοῦσιν. ὃ κ̓ ζημεῖον ὑπολαμβάνει ὡς ἴδιον τὸ τ῀ ἔδες.

πά. Αἱ μ̀ ἐν τ῀ λίθων διαφοραὶ, κ̓ δυνάμεις σχεδόν εἰσιν ἐν τούτοις

πϐ΄. Αἱ δ̓ τῆς γῆς ἐλάττονες μ̀, ἰδιώτεραι δέ.

πγ΄. Τὸ μ̀ [a] τήκεσϑ̓, καὶ ἀλλοιοῦσϑ̓, κ̓ πάλιν

──────────

[a] The Author now enters on an Account of the various Earths. The Differences of which are, indeed, very essential. It is to be observed, that he sets out in his usual Manner, perfectly, justly, and philosophically. The two great Characteristics of Earths, are their easy Diffusibility in Water, and Concretion and Induration on being separated from it, and their being fusible by Fire. The first of these Qualities essentially distinguishes them from most other Fossils. The other they have in common with Stones, and, indeed, with all other fossile Bodies whatever. It was impossible for this Author to have known this, unless he had had our Assistances. But we know by Experiments with powerful Burning-glasses, that all fossile Substances, as well as Earths, are fusible and vitrifiable, the Diamond itself not excepted, as has been observed more at large in its proper Place.

Earths, determinately speaking, are opake Bodies, diffusible by Water, and vitrifiable by extreme Heat, friable when dry, not inflammable, and generally insipid to the Taste. Not that these are certain, universal Characteristics, and li-

confonant to Reafon, as the upper Part is the dryer; for the Humidity of the other Surface hinders its receiving fo well the Particles of the Metals: For the fame Reafon alfo it does not perform its Office fo well in hot Weather as in colder, for in the hot it emits a kind of Humidity out of its Subftance, which runs all over it: This hinders the metalline Particles from adhering perfectly, and makes Miftakes in the Tryals. This Exfudation of a humid Matter is alfo common to many other Stones, among others, to thofe of which Statues are made; and this has been looked on as peculiar to the Statue

LXXXI. Thefe then, in general, are the Differences, and particular Qualities of Stones

LXXXII. Thofe of Earths are fewer, indeed, but they are alfo more peculiar.

LXXXIII. ᵃ Earth is fubject to be liquated,

---

ble to no Exceptions. Whatever may be the Cafe in the Vegetable and Animal Kingdoms, it is the Misfortune in the Study of foffile Bodies, that fuch has been the Confufion and Intermixture of their conftituent Particles at the general Deluge, that there are none fuch to be eftablifhed in it, for there are fo many heterogene Particles, of a thoufand different Kinds, mixed even with the fame Foffil in different Places, that there is no determining it to any Certainty, even in its manner of Variation from its pure State What I have given may pafs, however, for a general Character of what, in Treatifes of Foffils, we mean by the Word *Earths*; which may be afterwards diftinguifhed into *Clays, Ochres, Boles, Marles, Chalks,* and *Loams* Sand, and the common vegetable Mould, which fome give a Place in the Catalogues of Earths, have of right no Bufinefs among them; for the firft is only either a fmaller kind of Gravel, confifting of an infinite number of fmall Pebbles of different Shapes and Colours, or the conftituent Particles of the Stone of Strata or other Bodies

(116)

ἀποσκληρώσεϩ, κ) ταύτῃ ζυμβαίνᵉ· τήκεϳ μ̃ γὰρ
τοῖς χυλοῖς κ̀) ὀρυκϳοῖς, ὥσπερ ℂ ὁ λίθ⊕. μαλάτϳεϳ
ϳ, πλίνθυς τε ποιῦσιν, ὧν τάς τε ποικίλας, καὶ
τὰς ἄλλας τὰς ζυνϳιθεμϳίας. ἀπάσας ϳὲ πυρῦνϳες
κ) μαλάτϳονϳες, ποιῦσιν.

πδ΄. ᵇ Εἰ ϳ καὶ ὁ ὕελ⊕ ἐκ τ̃ ὑελίτιδ⊕, ὡς

---

accidentally loofe And the latter owes its prefent mode of Exiftence, in a great meafure, to putrified animal and vegetable Subftances of a thoufand Kinds, and is, diftinctly fpeaking, no genuine Foffil.

In order to the right underftanding what is meant by the calling any Subftance by either of the other Names, it may not be improper briefly to give their feveral Diftinctions, fo far as the general Uncertainty of the Foffile Kingdom will permit.

1 *Clays* are Earths compofed of very fine Parts, fmooth, heavy, not eafily mixing with Water, and when mixed, not readily fubfiding in it, compact, vifcid, and leaving a fatty Impreffion on the Tongue, foft while in the Stratum, and hardening by Fire into a kind of ftony Texture.

2 *Ochres* are ponderous earthy Subftances, more fat than Chalk, and lefs fo than Clay, readily diffufible in Water, and friable when dry, ftaining the Fingers in handling, and principally differing from the Boles, in that they are of a loofer Texture.

3. *Boles* are ponderous earthy Subftances, more fat than Chalk or Marle, but lefs fo than Clay, ponderous, of an aftringent Tafte, melting in the Mouth, ftaining the Fingers, and generally partaking more or lefs of the Nature of Iron, as indeed, in fome degree, do moft, if not all, the other Earths, but the Boles generally more than any

4. *Marles* are light friable Subftances, of a middle Nature, between Clay and Chalk, not fo fatty as the former, nor fo denfe as the latter, eafily diffufible in Water, and, when tafted, dry, infipid, and adhering to the Tongue.

5 *Chalks* are earthy Subftances, denfe, brittle, readily diffufible in Water, and quickly feparating themfelves from

altered from its original State and Confiftence, and afterwards indurated again. It will melt, as Stones, with fufible and foffile Subftances, and is foftened, and made into Bricks. Thefe are of various Kinds, and compofed in various Manners, but are all made by moiftening and burning.

LXXXIV. [b] But if Glafs be made, as fome af-

---

it by Subfidence, ftaining the Fingers in handling, and, in tafting, fticking to the Tongue

6 And *Loams* are earthy Bodies, of a denfe, rough Texture, confifting of clayey or ochreous Matter, with arenaceous Particles of various Figures, Sizes, and Colours, immerfed in and intimately mixed with it, probably, at the time of the univerfal Deluge.

Much more might be faid on this Occafion were this a proper Place for it, but this general and fuccinct Account of what is meant by the general Names of Clays, &c. may be fufficient for what is intended in this Place, which is only to give fomething of a determinate Idea of what is meant by the Words Chalk, Bole, &c. when there fhall be occafion hereafter to fay any of the Bodies defcribed by this Author is one or other of thefe fubftances

[b] All Earths, as I have before obferved, are vitrifiable by extreme degrees of Heat. Nothing is more certain, than that the Vitrification, or converting the Subftances of which Glafs is made, into that Form, is the Effect of the extreme Force of Fire; and that the beft fort of Glafs is that in the making of which Flints have been ufed, is a Truth as much known now, as it was in the days of *Theophraftus*.

The Things of which our Glafs is made are, Potafhes, (made in different Places from different Species of the Herb *Kali*, and other vegetable Subftances, by burning, and called by the *French Soude*, and by the *Italians Barilha* The common Pot-afhes are made from the *Kali Cochleatum majus*, but the fineft, from the *Kali Hifpanicum fupinum annuum, Sedi foliis brevibus*, figured and defcribed in the Memoirs of the Royal Acade-

τινές φασι, καὶ αὕτη πυρώσει γίνεται. ἰδιωτάτη δ' ἡ τῷ χάλικι μιγνυμένη. πρὸς γὰ τὸ τήκεσθαι καὶ μίγνυσθαι, καὶ δύναμιν ἔχει πλείτην, ὥστε τὸ κάλλει τῆς χρόας ποιεῖν διαφοράν.

πέ. Περὶ δὲ Κιλικίαν, ἐστὶ τίς ἡ ἑψητὴ γῆ, καὶ γίνεται γλισχρά. ταύτῃ δ' ἀλείφουσι τὰς ἀμπέλους ἀντὶ ἰξοῦ πρὸς τὰς ἶπας.

πς'. Εἴη δ' ἂν ς λαμβάνειν καὶ ταύτας τὰς διαφορὰς ὅσαι πρὸς τὴν ἀπολίθωσιν εὐφυεῖς· ἐπεὶ αἵ γε, τὰς τούτων ποιοῦσαι χυμοὺς διαφόρους, ἀλλή-

my of Sciences of *Paris*,) some stony arenaceous or crystalline Matter, as Sand, Flints, Crystal, or Marble, and Manganeze, a ferruginous Substance to which some add a small Quantity of pure Salt of Tartar These Ingredients are calcined into what the Workmen call Fritt, and afterwards run, by Violence of Fire, into Glass of different Colours and degrees of Purity, according to the different Ingredients.

The Glass of the Antients was, in the different Ages of the World, in different degrees of Purity and Excellence, according to the Ingredients of which they made it, which were Sand, Nitre, Flints, and Shells Sand was the first Ingredient ever used or thought of for the making Glass and for many Ages, there was even no other Sand used among the *Greeks* than that found clean washed on the Banks and in the Beds of Rivers, and this, from its Use, might very probably acquire the Name of Ὕαλος, or Glass-Sand

In the beginning of this Sentence, the other Copies of this Author have ἐστὶ. I have ventured to follow *Salmasius* in his most rational Opinion, that it was in the Original ἐστὶν, and a little afterwards to give

firm, of the *Uelitis*, a vitrifiable Sand, it owes its Production to the extreme Force of Fire: The best is that, in the making of which Flints have also been used; for besides that they melt and mix with the running Mass, they have a peculiar Excellence in the making the Glass, insomuch that they give the Differences in the clearness of the Colour

LXXXV. There is in *Cilicia* [b] a kind of Earth, which by boiling becomes tough and viscous, with which they cover the Vines instead of Birdlime, to preserve them from the Worms.

LXXXVI. It may also be proper to mention here the Earths which are naturally endued with a Quality of petrifying Substances immersed in them, since those which yield peculiar and different [c] Juices, have unquestionably some fixed and

---

χάλικι, for what has hitherto stood χάλκω according to *De Laet*, who very justly suspects, that Flints were much more likely to be made an Ingredient in Glass than Brass. And, indeed, when we consider the many Lacunæ and greater Errors in the Copies of this Author, we cannot wonder that such as these have been pass'd over, which were only Errors in a Letter or two

[b] The *Cilician* Earth, used as a Preserver of Vines from Insects, was of the Class of the harder Bitumens, which the Heat of Boiling-water would just bring to a proper Consistence for spreading over the Stocks of those Shrubs, and partly by entangling and smothering Insects that were climbing up, and partly by its driving them away by its Smell, it preserved the Buds from being destroyed

[c] The various Accounts we have of petrifying Earths and Waters, are all idle, erroneous, and imaginary, according to the ingenious and excellent Dr *Woodward*, who affirms, that even what has been reported so confidently of the petrifying Water of the Lake *Oireagh* in *Ireland*, one of the most famous Petrifying Springs on record, has been shewn, by a more

(120)

λων τιν' ἔχουσαι φύσιν· ὥσπερ καὶ αἱ τὰς τῶν φυτῶν [d].

πζ'. Ἀλλὰ μᾶλλον ἄν τις τὰς τοῖς χρώμασι διαριθμήσειε, οἷάπερ κ̀ οἱ γραφεῖς χρῶν[).

πή. Καὶ γὸ ἡ γένεσις τούτων, ὥσπερ ἐξ ἀρχῆς εἴπομεν, ἤτοι ξυρροῆς τινος, ἢ διηθήσεως γινομένης.

πθ'. Καὶ ἐνίαγε δὴ φαίνε[) πεπυρωμένα, κ̀ οἷον κατακεκαυμένα, οἷον κ̀ ἡ Σανδαράκη ὲ τὸ Ἀρρε-

---

accurate Enquiry and Tryals, not to be true, and that the petrified Wood brought thence, has been all of it lodged in the Earth at the bottom of that Lake at the time of the Deluge. If this be the Case here, it is, in all probability, in other Places too; and what gives it the better face of Probability is, that petrified Wood is is often found in the loose Strata of Gravel, &c. and lodged in Earth or Stone as in the Beds of these Waters. Some may imagine, from having seen the Effects of the dropping Well at Knaresborough, Rushbank, and several other Springs in Northamptonshire, Chedworth, and Norwich Springs in Gloucestershire, and many other petrifying Springs, as they are called in *England*, and elsewhere, that ——, denying things for which they have the Evidence of their senses. But such Persons are to be taught, that what they esteem Petrifactions, are no other than Incrustations of sparry, argillaceous, and other Matter, brought away with these Waters in their Passage through the Strata, and settling from them again. And that there is great Difference between changing the very Substance, and only covering the Surface of a Body. These Petrifactions, as they are called, being no other than Precipitations of Matter too heavy to be longer sustained in the Water, and which, being very fine, adapts itself to every Prominence and Cavity of the Body it settles upon, and exactly assumes its Shape. The first Process in these Ope-

peculiar Properties, and are diſtinct Kinds; as are also thoſe which ſupply Nouriſhment to Plants [d]

LXXXVII. Nor ought thoſe to be leſs conſidered which are ſingular and remarkable in their Colours, and for that Reaſon uſed by Painters.

LXXXVIII. The Production of theſe, as was obſerved in the Beginning of this Treatiſe, is from the mere Afflux or Percolation of their conſtituent Particles.

LXXXIX. Some of theſe ſeem burnt, and to have ſuffered Changes by means of Fire, as [e] Sandarach, Orpiment, and others of that Kind; all of

---

tions of Nature forms only an extremely thin Cruſt over the Body, on which there after ſettle at Times many more, often to a Cruſt of conſiderable Thickneſs in the whole, but always giving evident Proofs of the Manner in which it was ſucceſſively formed, by the Number of thin Strata it is compoſed of.

[d] Vegetable Mould, I have before obſerved, is no genuine Foſſil.

[e] Orpiment and Sandarach have been ſpoken of in general already; they are found in different degrees of Purity and Beauty. In ſome Places, inſtead of the fine foliaceous Flakes, or ſhining Glebes, in which they are dug in moſt of the Mines, they are taken up impure, ill colour'd and in form of a coarſe Powder, the yellow looking more like dirty Fragments of common Brimſtone, and the red like duſty pieces of a bad Bole, than like what they really are. Theſe are, however, purchaſed by our Painters for Cheapneſs, and they ſay, with proper Management, make as good Colours as the finer Pieces, though, in their Barrels, they look more like Aſhes than the beautiful Subſtances they really are. Theſe are from ſome part of Germany. And if the Orpiments and Sandarachs which happened to come in Theophraſtus's way, were of this Kind, there is nothing ſtrange in his ſuppoſing them to have been acted upon by ſubterranean Fires.

νικὸν, ϗ τὰ ἄλλα τὰ τοιαῦτα. πάντα δ', ὡς ἁπλῶς εἰπεῖν, ἀπὸ τῆ ἀναθυμιάσεως, ταῦτα ϝ ξηρᾶς ϗ καπνώδες. ἃ ρίσκε] δὴ πάντα ἐν τοῖς μετάλλοις τοῖς ἀργυρείοις τε καὶ χρυσείοις· ἔνια ϳ ϗ ἐν τοῖς χαλκωρυχείοις.

ί. Οἷον ᶠ Ἀρρενικὸν, Σανδαράκη, Χρυσοκόλλα, ᵍ Μίλτ⊙, Ὤχρα, Κύαν⊙, ἐλάχιστ⊙ ϳ ἔτ⊙,

---

ᶠ The Ochre here meant is the common yellow Kind. A Confirmation that the ἀρρενικὸν of the Antients was Orpiment, and not a white Arsenick, as some have erroneously judged, is this Passage of this Author, where he says, It is, when powdered, of the Colour of the yellow Ochre

The Yellow Ochre of many Parts of this Kingdom is excellent for the Use of Painters, and some of it finer than any in the World It is found of two Kinds, the one in great plenty, constituting, in many Places, whole Strata of very considerable Thickness This is the most common, but is coarse, and often mixed with arenaceous and other heterogene Matter in different Quantities. The other Kind is found in the perpendicular Fissures of other Strata. This is not common, nor to be had in any great plenty, but is ever of a glorious Colour, and perfectly pure, and crumbles between the Fingers into an impalpable Powder As all the Matter which composes it must have been extremely fine and subtle, or it never could have got into those Places, into which there was no way for it, but thro' the Pores of the solid Strata I know not whether our Painters are acquainted with this Kind, but it must, as *Woodward* has observed, be very much preferable to the common ones for their Use, because of its Fineness, and it might be had in some Quantity on searching the proper Places I remember to have seen much of it in different Places about *Mendip* Hills in *Somersetshire*, from whence I brought the Specimens in my possession

ᵍ Reddle, or Red Ochre, is as common and as good in

them, however, plainly speaking, owe their present Form to the Exhalation of their more humid Parts; and these, in particular, seem to have been dried, and, as it were, smoaked. They are found in Mines of Gold and Silver, and some in those of Copper also.

XC. Of this kind are ᶠ Orpiment, Sandarach, Chryfocolla, ᵍ Reddle, Ochre, and the *Lapis Armenus*, but

---

England as the Yellow; it is, like that, generally found itself forming Strata, but sometimes of a glorious Colour and extreme Fineness, in Fissures of other Strata. I have a Specimen of some from the Forest of *Dean* in *Gloucestershire*, very little inferior to the Sort brought from the Island of *Ormuz* in the *Persian* Gulph, and so much valued and used by our Painters under the Name of *Indian* Red. It is, indeed, so like, both in Colour and Quality, that it is used for it, as the People employed in taking it up informed me, and sent to *London* to be sold under its Name. On comparing it with some of the true *Persian* kind, which I had from the *East-Indies*, I find it of a paler Colour, but of a much finer Texture; and therefore, upon the whole, perhaps not less valuable.

Misunderstandings of *Pliny*, occasioned by Errors in the Copies, have been the Occasion of some very unlucky Errors about the μίλτος of the *Greeks*, which has been concluded, from what he has been supposed to have said, to be Cinnabar, which they called also *Minium*. The Passage which has given Occasion to these Mistakes stands in most Copies thus, *Milton vocant Græci Minium, quidam Cinnabari*, which seems an absolute Affirmation of this, but is, in reality, no other than a double Error, in the Words, and in the Pointing. And what *Pliny* meant to have said is evidently no other than this, *Rubricam Milton Græci vocant, & minium Cinnabari*. The *Greeks* call Reddle *Miltos*, and *Minium Cinnabar*, which is exactly the Truth. And the Passage, as thus restored by *Salmasius*, stands accordingly, *Jam enim Trojanis temporibus rubrica in honore erat, qui naves ea commendat, alias circa pi-*

κ੍ਰ κατ' ἐλάχιςα. τ̄ δ' ἄλλων μέν εἰσι ῥάβδοι, τὴν δ' Ὤχραν ἀθρόαν πῶς φασιν εἶναι. Μίλτον δε παντοδαπὴν, ὥςε εἰς τὰ ἀνδρείκελα χρῆαζ τὰς γραφεῖς. κ੍ਰ Ὤχραν ἀντ' Ἀρρενικᾶ, Διὰ τὸ μηδὲν τῇ χρόα Διαφέρειν, δοκεῖν δέ.

ιά. Ἀλλὰ Μίλτ̄ τε κ੍ਰ Ὤχρας ἐςὶν ἐνιαχῦ μέταλλα. κ੍ਰ κατ ταῦτα, καθάπερ ἐν Καππαδοκίᾳ, κ੍ਰ ὀρύτ[εζ] πολλή. χαλεπὸν δ τοῖς μεγάλλοις φασὶν εἶναι τὸ πνίγεαζ. ταχὺ γὰρ κᾳ ἐν ὀλίγῳ τᾶτο ποιεῖν.

ιβ'. Βελτίςη δ δοκεῖ μίλτ⊙ ἡ Κέα εἶναι. (γίνονται γ̄ πλείυς.) ἡ μ̄ ȣν ἐκ τ̄ μεγάλλων, ἐπειδὴ κ੍ਰ τὰ σιδήρεια ἔχει [h] μίλτον.

───────────────

fturas, pigmentaque rarus Milton *vocant* Græci, minium*que* Cinnabari. Homer, speaking of the *Greci in* Ships, has Νῆας μιλτοπαρηυς and it is impossible he should mean by it, that they were stained with the *Minium,* or Cinnabar, which was not known till after his Time, as we shall see by this Author's Account of it hereafter. Cinnabar was originally the *Indian* Name of the Gum we now call *Sanguis Draconis*, and was given to this other Substance (called also *Minium,*) from its Resemblance to that in Colour.

[h] Reddle always contains in it more or less of Iron, and there is one kind of it called Smitt in *England,* which is sometimes so rich, as to be worth working for that Metal, and have the Name of an Iron Ore. What this Author observes, of its being better in the Reddle Pits than in Iron Mines, is contrary to what we find now in *England.* The Reddle I just before have mentioned, as sometimes sold in *London* under the Name of *Indian* Red, is much

this laſt is ſcarce, and found only in ſmall Quantites; whereas there are ſometimes whole Veins of the others. Ochre is ſaid to be found generally heaped together; and Reddle ſcattered, as it were, every way. Painters uſe this Reddle in their Pictures, as alſo Ochre, inſtead of Orpiment, for when powder'd they ſcarce at all differ in Colour, however different they appear in the Maſs.

XCI. There are alſo in ſome Places peculiar Pits of Reddle and Ochre, as in *Cappadocia*, from whence they are taken in vaſt Quantities. But in theſe Pits, it is ſaid, the Labourers are in danger of Suffocation, which unhappy Accident ſometimes comes on very ſuddenly.

XCII. The beſt Reddle, for there are many Kinds, is thought to be that of *Cea*, and particularly that which is taken from the Reddle Pits; for it is alſo ſometimes found in [h] Iron Mines.

---

the fineſt I have ever ſeen, and that was not from a Reddle Pit, but from among the Iron Ore in the Foreſt of *Dean*. I have ſeen the Pits peculiarly worked for this Subſtance in *Derbyſhire* and *Staffordſhire*, and have of the Reddle from them, which is good, but much inferior to that of the Foreſt of *Dean* in all reſpects. And, indeed, Reaſon informs us that it always naturally muſt be ſo, for it muſt, as I before obſerved, neceſſarily be vaſtly finer in the Fiſſures of Strata, than where it conſtitutes Strata itſelf. And as all Reddle owes its Colour, which is its Value, to Iron, it muſt naturally have moſt of it, when neareſt the largeſt Quantities of that Metal. I can therefore ſee no Reaſon for that of the Pit's being eſteemed the beſt by the Antients, unleſs they valued it for its Texture and Conſiſtence. Then, indeed, that muſt be preferred, as it is the moſt compact and denſe, the other being ever looſer and more crumbly.

(126)

ιγ'. Ἀλλὰ κ̀ ἡ [1] Λημνία, ἣν καλοῦσιν Σινωπικήν· αὕτη δ᾽ ἐςὶν ἡ Καππαδοκική. καὶ ἄγεται δ᾽ εἰς Σινώπlω. ἐν ᾗ τῇ Λήμνῳ μεταλλούε]) καθ᾽ αὑτlώ.

ιδ'. Ἔςι ὴ αὐτῆς γνή τεία k. ἡ μ̀ ἐρυθρὰ σφό-

---

[1] There were among the Antients two Earths of *Lemnos* well known and in common Use, though to different Purposes. These Distinctions have been since lost, and that Loss has caused us a great deal of Confusion. These two were distinguish'd by the Names of *Terra Lemnia*, and *Rubrica Lemnia*, Γῆ Λημνία and Μίλτος Λημνία, the *Lemnian* Reddle, and *Lemnian* Earth. The first of these was used by Painters, as it was taken out of the Pit, the second was first made into Cakes, and sealed with great Ceremonies, and was in very high esteem in Medicine. I shall be the more particular on these Earths, as it will naturally lead to a better understanding of some other of the Earths now much in use in Medicine, at least the Names of which are so. The great Occasion of the Errors about the *Lemnian* Earths, is the Mistake of *Pliny*, in confounding them together, as he evidently has done, not distinguishing the medicinal sealed Earth of that Place, from the Reddle used by Painters. The sealed Earth was esteemed sacred, and the Priests alone were suffered to meddle with it. They mixed it with Goat's Blood, made the Impression of a Seal upon it, and it was, therefore, called σφραγίς, and *Sphragis* by the *Latins*, ἡ δὲ Λημνία λεγομένη γῆ ἐςὶν ἐκ τινος ὑπο ὁμε ἀνθώδε, ἀ ἀφερομένη κ̀ μιγομένη αἵματι αἰγείω, ἢν οἱ ἐκεῖ ἄνθρωποι ἀπλάσσο], κ̀ σφραγιζόμενοι εἰκόνι αἰγὸς, σφραγίδα καλοῦσιν, *Dioscorides*. This, therefore, was the Sealed Earth of *Lemnos*, the Earth used in Medicine, and called by the Physicians *Lemnian* Earth. The hand the Priests had in the making it up, got it the Name of Sacred Earth, Γῆ ἱερά. And this seems to be the very same with the true *Terra Lemnia* used at this time; which is a fat unctuous Clay, of a pale red Colour, made up in Cakes of about half an Ounce weight, sometimes less, and brought from *Lemnos*, and many other parts of the *Turkish* Dominions: This we

XCIII. There are beside these also, the [1] *Lemnian Reddle*, and the *Sinopic*, as it is commonly called; but it is dug in *Cappadocia*, and thence carried to *Sinope*. There are particular Pits in *Lemnos*, in which nothing but the Earth is dug.

XCIV. There are three kinds of the [k] *Sinopic*;

---

now call *Terra Lemnia Rubra*, by way of distinction from a white Earth, less unctuous and more astringent than the red, which is dug in *Lemnos* only. And we have sometimes, beside these, an unsealed Earth from the same Place, which is yellowish, with blackish Specks, and has this Advantage of the other, that we are sure it is genuine, for we are sensible they are too often counterfeited.

These were the *Terræ Lemniæ* used in Medicine. The *Rubrica Lemnia* was a kind of Reddle of a firm Consistence and deep red Colour, dug in the same Place, but never made into any Form or sealed, but purchased in the rough Glebes by Artificers of many kinds, who had Uses for it in Colouring. That *Pliny* confounds these two Substances is to be seen in this Passage *Rubricæ genus in ea... maximè intelligi. Quidam secundæ auctoritatis, palmam cum Lemniæ dabant. Minio proxima hæc est, multum corporis celebrata, cum insula in qua nascitur, nec nisi signata venundabatur, unde & Sphragidem appellavere.* Where it is evident, that he thought the *Lemnian* Reddle was the Substance sealed and called *Sphragis*, or Sealed Earth. But that they were not the same, and the Earth, and not the Reddle was the Substance which was seal'd, is evident from *Galen*, l. 1. de Antidotis, Καθαπερ επι Λημνιας γης κ̓ μίλε, καλ̓ ῶ δ᾽ αυτην αμεινον ὁ μίλιος, αλλα γην ἐςι γαρ τις Λημνια μιξις ἐν τη Λημνῳ, γενομενη προς αλλας χρειας επιτηδειος, ἡ μη τις ἀς᾽ ἡ καλυμενη Λημνια σφ̔ραγις.

[k] The *Sinopic* Earth, which we know at present is the first Kind mentioned by this Author, the other two we are wholly unacquainted with, though among the Antients they were much in esteem with Painters. Our *Rubrica Sinopica* is a dense, heavy, firm Substance, of a deep red Colour, staining the Fingers in handling, and of a styptic astringent Taste. *Tournefort* imagines it a native *Crocus*

δρα, ἡ δ᾽ ἔκλακ(ος), ἡ δὲ μέση. ταύτην αὐτάρκη καλῶμεν, διὰ τὸ μὴ μίγνυσθαι. τὰς δὲ ἑτέρας μιγνύουσι.

ιέ. Γίνεται δὲ ἐκ τῆς Ὤχρας κατακαιομένης. ἄλλη χείρων· τὸ δὲ εὕρημα Κυδίου (συνειδὲ γὰρ σκεῦ(ος), ὥς φασι, καταικαυθέντ(ος) τινὸς πανδοχείου, τὴν Ὤχραν ἰδὼν ἡμίκαυστον καὶ πεφοινιγμένην.

ις'. Τιθέασι δ' εἰς τὰς καμίνους χύτρας κενὰς περιπλάσαντες πηλῷ. Ὀπτῶσι γὰρ διάπυροι γινόμεναι. Ὅσῳ δ᾽ ἂν μᾶλλον πυρωθῶσι, τοσούτῳ μᾶλλον μελαντέραν, καὶ ἀνθρακωδεστέραν ποιοῦσι, μαρτυρεῖ δ᾽ ἂν ἡ χνεσις αὐτό· δόξειε γὰρ τὸ ὑπὸ πυρὸς ἅπαντα ταῦτα μεταβάλλειν· εἴπερ ὁμοίαν ἢ παραπλησίαν δεῖ τὴν ἐνταῦθα τῇ φυσικῇ κομίζειν¹.

Martis, and certain it is, that it owes its Colour, at least, to that Metal.

It is dug at this Time, as it was in that of *Theophrastus*, in *Cappadocia*, and carried to *Sinope* for Sale, from whence it has its Name, and from whence *Sinopis* became afterwards a general Name for the Red Ochres. Μίλτος εἶδο, ἐρυθρὸν Σινώπιδος, *Hesychius*, and so many others. If the present Esteem for this Substance was greater than it is, as indeed I can on Experience affirm it ought to be, it might be had, I believe, in many other Places beside *Cappadocia*. I have
some

of a deep Red, another of a whitish Colour, and the other of a middle Colour between the other two, which is called the pure simple Kind, because it is used without mixing, whereas they mix the others.

XCV. There is also a kind of this made of Ochre, by burning, but it is not nearly so good as the others. The making this was an Invention of *Cydias*, who took the Hint of it, as is said, from observing, in a House which was on fire, that some Ochre which was there, when half burnt, assumed a red Colour.

XCVI. The way of making the factitious is this. They put the Ochre into new earthen Vessels, which they cover with Clay and set in Furnaces, and these, as they grow hot, heat also the Ochre, and the greater degree of Fire they give, the deeper and more strongly purple the Matter becomes. The Origin of the native Kinds seems to testify that this Method is not irrational, for all these seem to have suffered Changes by the action of Fire. From whence we may rationally conclude, that this way of making the factitious, is either of the same kind, or at least very analagous to that used by Nature for the Production of the genuine[1].

---

some of it perfectly fine, which was dug in the *New Jersey* in *America*, where it is frequently found in digging at about 15 or 20 Feet deep, and is called, I suppose from its Colour and staining the Hands, Blood-stone. It was originally used, not only in Painting, but in Medicine; and though now disused, and not known in the Shops, deserves to be brought into Use again, being a much better Astringent, as I have found by repeated Tryals of that from *America*, than any of the Earths now in use.

[1] The making a Red Ochre from the Yellow by burning

ιζ. Ἔστι δ᾽ ὥσπερ κ̀ Μίλτος, ἡ μ̀ αὐτόματος, ἡ δ̀ τεχνική[11].

ιή. Καὶ Κύανος, ὁ μ̀ αὐτοφυής· ὁ δ̀, σκευαστὸς, ὥσπερ ἐν Αἰγύπτῳ· γένη γὸ Κυανῦ τρία· ἡ Αἰγύπτιος, κ̀ Σκύθης, ἐ τρίτος ὁ Κύπριος· βέλτιστος δ᾽ ὁ Αἰγύπτιος εἰς τὰ ἄκρατα λειώματα. ὁ δ̀ Σκύθης, εἰς τὰ ὑδαρέστερα. Σκευαστὸς δ᾽ ὁ Αἰγύπτιος· κ̀ οἱ γράφοντες τὰ περὶ τὺς Βασιλεῖς, κ̀ τῦτο γράφυσι, τίς πρῶτος Βασιλεὺς ἐποίησε τεχνητὸν Κυανὸν, μιμησάμενος τ᾽ αὐτοφυῆ.

---

is as well known, and as much practised among the People who deal in Colours for painting now, as it was in the Time of this Author. I cannot but observe, however, that his calling this a *Sinopis*, is a Proof of what I have before observed, that that Word became a Name for all the Substances of the Red Ochre kind. As to what this Author observes, of the native Red Ochres owing their Colour to Fire, it is very certain, that most of them shew no Marks of ever having been acted on by that Element. And we know very well, that the ferrugineous Particles which can make the Matter red in burning, can also impart that Colour to it without the assistance of Fire. Notwithstanding which, it must be allowed, that there are some of these red Substances; and not only these, but some other Bodies, particularly some of the Hæmatites kind, which seem, even in their native Beds, to carry evident Marks of their having been wrought on and changed by Fire, though it is not easy to say, how or when it should have happened.

[11] The factitious *Sinopis* just mentioned, I have observed, was no other than a factitious Reddle, properly speaking, and what the Author here mentions, was probably another Kind, made from some other Species of Yellow Ochre,

XCVII. The Reddle also is of two Kinds, the native, and the factitious [11].

XCVIII. There is also, beside the native *Lapis Armenus*, a factitious Kind made in *Egypt*. There are, indeed, three different Sorts of this, the *Egyptian*, the *Scythian*, and the *Cyprian* [m], of which the *Egyptian* is the best for clear strong Paintings, and the *Scythian* for the fainter. The *Egyptian* is factitious, and the Historians, who write the Annals of the Kings of that Nation, think it a thing worthy a Place in their Histories, which King of *Egypt* was the Inventer of the artificial *Cæruleum* in Imitation of the native.

---

and called Reddle, from its being of a pale red, and resembling that of the common native Red Ochre, as the other was called factitious *Sinopis*, from its being of a deeper, and resembling the genuine *Sinopis* of *Cappadocia*.

[n] I have, in another Place, observed the Confusion which has arisen from *Pliny*'s confounding the Cyanus Gem with the Cyanus Paint, or *Lapis Armenus*. We have a great Instance of this Error in his Translation of this Passage of our Author, which he has given the Sense of, but has rendered the Whole perfectly unintelligible, by saying all this of the Cyanus Gem, which it is most evident *Theophrastus* says of the *Lapis Armenus*, or Cyanus Paint. There can be no question but that this Author is here treating of this Substance, the Cyanus Paint, or *Lapis Armenus*, and not the *Lapis Lazuli*, as he has done with the Gems long since; and is now treating of the Earths, and particularly those used in Painting, and his Description of the Use of it makes it so notoriously plain, that it is astonishing *Pliny* could mistake him. The Passage in *Pliny* is (speaking of the Cyanus Gem) *Optima Scythica, dein Cypria, postremo Ægyptia. Adulteratur maximè tincturâ, idque in gloria regis Ægyptii ascribitur, qui primus eam tinxit, dividitur autem & hæc in mares faminasque. inest ei aliquando & aureus pulvis, &c.*

ιθ'. Δῶρά τε πέμπεσθαι παρ' ἄλλων τε καὶ ἐκ Φοινίκης· φόρον Κυανοῦ, τοῦ μὲν ἀπύρου, τοῦ δὲ πεπυρωμένου.

ρ'. ᵐΦασὶ δ' οἱ τὰ φάρμακα τρίβοντες, τὸν μὲν Κυανὸν ἐξ ἑαυτοῦ ποιεῖν χρώματα τέτταρα. τὸ μὲν πρῶτον, ἐκ τῶν λεπτοτάτων λευκότατον· τὸ δὲ δεύτερον, ἐκ τῶν παχυτάτων μελάντατον.

ρα'. Ταῦτά τε δὴ τέχνῃ γίνεται, καὶ ἔτι τὸ ψιμύθιον. τίθεται γὰρ μόλιβδος ὑπὲρ ὄξυς ἐν πίθοις. ὅταν δὲ λάβῃ πάχος ἡλίκον πλῆθος, (λαμβάνει δὲ μάλιστα ἐν ἡμέραις δέκα) τότ' ἀνοίγουσιν· εἶτ' ἀπο-

---

ᵐ The Colours, of different degrees of Deepness, which were prepared from this Substance, were separated by means of Water: The Method of preparing them was, by beating the Matter to Powder, and putting that in a large quantity of Water, and saving, in different Vessels, that which subsided at different Times, the heavier part, consisting of larger Particles, sinking almost immediately, and the lighter, which consisted of much smaller and finer, not till after a considerable Time. These different Quantities of Colour that had subsided at the different Times, were then separately ground to a proper Fineness, and kept as different Colours for Use. And this is the Meaning of the λεπτοτάτων and παχυτάτων of our Author, and *Crassiorem tenuioremve* of *Pliny*. Which some, who imagined they were talking of the Degree of Colour, and not of the Fineness and Coarseness of the Particles of the Matter, could not bring themselves to understand. Indeed, in many of the Passages complained of as unintelligible in the Antients, the Obscurity has been more owing to the wrong Apprehension of the Commentators, than the Perplexity of the Authors.

XCIX. Presents are also made to great Persons in some Places of this Substance, as well that which has passed the Fire as that which has not, and the *Phœnicians* pay their Tribute in it

C.ᵐ People who prepare Colours say also, that the *Lapis Armenus* of itself makes four different ones; the two Extremes of which are, first, that which consists only of its finest Particles, and is very pale, and the other, that which consists of its largest, and is extremely deep.

CI. But these are the Works of Art, as is also Ceruse ⁿ, to make which, Lead is placed in earthen Vessels over sharp Vinegar, and after it has acquired some thickness of a kind of Rust, which it commonly does in about ten Days, they open the Vessels, and scrape it off, as it were, in a kind of Foul-

---

ⁿ We have three or four different Methods of making Ceruse now used among us, but all are of the same Kind with this of *Theophrastus*, and are the Effect of Vinegar on Lead. It is by some made by infusing Filings of Lead in strong Vinegar, which in twelve or fourteen Days will almost entirely dissolve them, and leave a very good Ceruse at the bottom of the Vessel. Others make it, by plunging thin Plates of the same Metal into Vinegar, and placing them in a gentle Heat, these Plates will be, in about ten Days or less, covered with a white Rust, which is to be scraped off, and the Plates plunged into the Vinegar again, and so scraped at Times till they are wholly eaten in pieces: All the different Scrapings are afterwards ground to Powder together and kept for Use. And others make it, by putting Vinegar into an earthen Vessel, then covering it closely with a plate of Lead, and setting it in the Sun in hot Weather, and this Plate will, in about ten Days, be dissolved and precipitated in form of Ceruse to the bottom of the Vessel.

ξύωσιν ὥσπερ ἱδρῶτά τινα ἀπ' αὐτό, ἢ πάλιν (τιθέασι) ἢ πάλιν ἕως ἂν καταναλώσωσι. τὸ δ' ἀπο-
ξυόμβρον, ἐν τριχθέρι τρίβυσι, ἢ ἐφθῶσιν ἀεί. τὸ ἢ
ἔσχατον ὑφιςάμβρον ἐςι τὸ ψιμύθιον.

ρϛ'. Παραπλησίως ἢ ἢ ὁ ἰὸς γίνε). Χαλκὸς ϟ
ἐρυθρὸς, ὑπὲρ τρυγὸς τίθε), ἢ ἀποξυέ) τὸ ἐπι-
γινόμβρον. ὅτω ἐπιφαίνε) τιθέμβροͦ[n].

ρζ'. Γίνε) ἢ ἢ Κιννάβαρι· τὸ μ̃ αὐτοφυὲς, τὸ
ἢ, κατ' ἐργασίαν[o]. αὐτοφυὲς μ̃, τὸ πρὶ Ἰϐηρίαν,

---

[n] Our Manner of making Verdigrese is as like this of the Antients, as that of our making Ceruse, and it is very evident, that both the one and the other have been handed down from very early Ages to us. The Manner in which we make it is this. The Pressings of Grapes are, when taken from the Press, spread on Hurdles, and laid in the Sun to dry, after they have lain in this Manner two or three Days, and are pretty well dried, they are made into a Paste with Wine, and left to ferment; afterwards, while in a state of Fermentation, they are made into Balls, and again laid in Wine till thoroughly wetted with it, and then placed in proper Vessels at a little distance over the Wine, and shut up together in this manner for near a Fortnight, after which they smell very strong and pungent, and are in a Condition to extract the Rust from Copper, they are then beaten together into a Paste, and laid, *Stratum super Stratum*, with thin Plates of Copper, on wooden Bars in the same Vessels; and in a Week or ten Days the Verdigrese is formed. The Plates are then taken out, and wrapt in linnen Cloths dipped in Wine, and laid for three Weeks in a Cellar. After which the Verdigrese is scraped off for Use.

[o] The Antients, we find, had what they called the na-

ness, they then place the Lead over the Vinegar again, repeating over and over the same Method of scraping it, till it is wholly dissolved; what has been scraped off they then beat to Powder, and boil for a long time; and what at last subsides to the bottom of the Vessel is the Ceruse.

CII. In a manner also, something resembling this, is Verdigrease made, for Copper is placed over the Lees of Wine, and the Rust which it acquires by this means is taken off for Use. And it is by this means that the Rust which appears is produced [n].

CIII. There are also two kinds of Cinnabar, the one native, the other factitious [o], the native, which

---

tive and factitious Cinnabar as well as we, their native Cinnabar was the same with ours, but the factitious very widely different. Theirs was, we see, no other than a Preparation of a fine shining arenaceous Substance, which was the *Sal Atticum Romanorum* injudiciously confounded by *Imperius* with the *Ochra Attica* of the Antients, whereas ours is a Substance formed, by the Art of Chemistry, of Quicksilver and Sulphur, into a dense heavy Mass, of a bright red, marked with shining silvery Streaks.

The native Cinnabar of the Antients and of the Moderns are, however, the same, and theirs, as well as ours, was a dense heavy mineral Substance, of a shining red Colour, from which Quicksilver was extracted. This Substance was also called *Minium*, and, in After-times, becoming subject to Adulterations with Lead Ore calcined to a Redness, after the two Names had long been used in common, the Word *Minium* became at last appropriated to the calcined Lead Ore only, and the Cinnabar was used only to signify what we now understand by it, the Substance from which Quicksilver was to be extracted.

The Word Cinnabar κιννάβαρι, however, among the old Writers in Medicine, frequently is used to signify a Thing of a very different Kind, a vegetable Juice, called by us

σκληρὸν σφόδρα κ̣ λιθῶδες· ὃ τὸ ἐν Κόλχοις. τῶν δέ φασιν εἶναι κρημνῶν. ἐνκαταβάλλυσι τοξεύοντες. τὸ δὲ κατ' ἐργασίαν ὑπὲρ Ἐφέσυ μικρὸν ἐξ ἑνὸς τόπυ. μόνον δ' ἐστὶν ἄμμος, ἣν συλλέγυσι λαμπυρίζυσαν, καθάπερ ὁ κόκκος· ταύτην δὲ τρίψαντες ὅλως ἐν ἀγγείοις λιθίνοις λειοτάτην πλύνυσιν ἐν χαλκοῖς, μικρὸν ἐν κάλοις. τὸ δ' ὑφιστάμενον πάλιν λαβόντες, πλύνυσι κ̣ τρίβυσιν. ἐν ᾧπερ ἐστὶ τὸ ῥ

Dragons-blood, and long idly believed to be really the Blood of Dragons. This generally was, however, called Κιννάβαρι Ἰνδικὸν, from its Country, to diſtinguiſh it from the other, or mineral Cinnabar, γίνεται δὲ ἐν αὐτῇ κ̣ Κιννάβαρι τὸ λεγόμενον Ἰνδικὸν, ἀπὸ τῶν δένδρων ὡ, δάκρυ συναγόμενον, *Dioſcorides.*

This Cinnabar they therefore knew as a perfectly diſtinct Subſtance, though called by the ſame Name. And the mineral native Cinnabar, the thing here ſpoken of, was, we find, a hard ſtony Subſtance. Ours is a compact weighty Body, found ſometimes pure, and ſometimes incorporated with different other Subſtances, or containing other Subſtances incorporated with it.

The pure Cinnabar is generally of a bright red, ſometimes deeper, ſometimes paler, but commonly ſparkling or gloſſy; ſome is found of a deeper and duſkier Colour in the Maſs, but becomes of a fine Red when rubbed to Powder. And ſome of it reſembles the Hæmatites of ſome Kinds.

When incorporated with other Subſtances, it is chiefly found in Spar, or in looſe, arenaceous or ſparry Stones, ſometimes, but much more rarely, in clayey Earth, and ſometimes in a talky Matter, greyiſh, or bluiſh, or whitiſh.

is found in *Spain*, is hard and stony; as is also that brought from *Colchis*, which they say is produced there in Rocks and on Precipices, from which they get it down with Darts and Arrows. The factitious is from the Country a little above *Ephesus*; it is but in small Quantities, and is had only from one Place. It is only a Sand, shining like Scarlet, which they collect, and rub to a very fine Powder, in Vessels of Stone only, and afterwards wash in other Vessels of Brass, or sometimes of Wood. What subsides they go to work on again, rubbing it and washing it as before. And in this Work there is much Art to be used; for from an equal Quantity of the Sand some will make a large Quantity of the

---

It frequently holds incorporated with it, beside Quick-silver, Gold, Silver, sparry and marcasitical Bodies, and sometimes Lead.

It is found in *Hungary, Bohemia, Saxony, Spain, France, Italy,* and the *East-Indies*, but no where in greater plenty then about *Rosenburg* in *Hungary*, where it is found chiefly in a whitish sparry Stone on the sides of the Hills, and is gathered by the poor People, after it has been cleared and uncovered by Rains. The purer native Cinnabar has been used to be much esteemed both by the Painters and in Medicine, but our factitious kind equalling it in Beauty, and being much cheaper, has banished it from among the Painters. And it were to be wish'd the Case were the same in Medicine, for the Dose may be much better ascertained in the factitious, than the native, which we can never be sure of as to its exact degree of Purity, and which may also contain other mineral Substances, which we have no Intent of giving, mixed and incorporated with it. That of *Hungary*, however, is what always ought to be kept for internal Use (if it be to be so used) as it is commonly more pure than that of any other Place.

τέχνης. οἱ μ̃ γ̃ ἐκ ξ̃ ἴσυ πολὺ ϖἐιποιῦσιν· οἱ δ̃, ὀλίγον, ἢ ὐθέν· ἀλλὰ ϖλύσμαϳι ἐπάνω χρῶνϳ), ἐν ϖρὸς ἐν ἀλείφονϳες. γίνεϳ δ̃ τὸ μ̃ ὑςάμϕνον κάτω Κιννάϐαρι· τὸ δ᾽ ἐπάνω κ̃ ϖλεῖον, ϖλύσμα.

ρδ΄. Καϳαδεῖξαι δέ φασι κ̃ εὑρεῖν τὴν ἐργασίαν, Καλλίαν τινα Ἀθηναῖον ἐκ τ̃ ἀργυρείων. ὃς οἰόμψϙ̃ ἔχειν τ̃ ἄμμον χρυσίον, διὰ τὸ λαμπυρίζειν, ἐπραγματδύετο κ̃ ζυνέλεγψ. ἐπεὶ δ̃ ἤσθεϳο ὅτι οὐκ ἔχι, τὸ δ̃ τ̃ ἄμμυ κάλλ@̃ ἐθαύμαζε διὰ τὴν χρόαν, ὕτως ἐπὶ τ̃ ἐργασίαν ἦλθε ταύτην. ὐ ϖαλαιὸν δ᾽ ἐςίν· ἀλλὰ ϖἐὶ ἔτη μάλις᾽ ἐνενήκονϳα εἰς ἄρχονϳα Πραξίϐυλον Ἀθήνησι.

ρε΄. Φανερὸν δ᾽ ἐκ τύτων, ὅτι μιμεῖται τὴν φύσιν ἡ τέχνη, τὰ δ̃ ἴδια ϖοιεῖ. κ̃ τύτων τὰ μ̃ χρήσεως χάριν, τὰ δ̃ μόνον φανϳασίας, ὥσπερ τὰς ἀλιπές. ἔνια δ᾽ ἴσως ἀμφοῖν ὥσπερ χυτὸν ἄργυρον [p] ἔςι γὰρ τις χρεία κ̃ τύτυ. ϖοιεῖται δ᾽ ὅταν τι (Κιννάϐαρι)

---

[p] We have now many ways of extracting the Quickſilver from Cinnabar, but all by the Aſſiſtance of Fire Where the Mineral is rich, the common way is by a kind of Deſtillation *per deſcenſum* in this Manner· After beating it to Powder, it is put into narrow-neck'd earthen Veſſels, which are ſtopped with bundles of Moſs crambed pretty hard into them Theſe are then turned bottom upwards, and their Necks, thus ſtopped, let into the Mouths of other

Powder, and others very little, or none at all. The washing they use is very light and superficial, and they wet it every time separately and carefully. That which at last subsides is the Cinnabar, and that which swims above in much larger quantity is only the superfluous Matter of the Washing

CIV. It is said, that one *Callias*, an *Athenian*, who belonged to the Silver Mines, invented and taught the making this artificial Cinnabar. He had carefully got together a great quantity of this Sand, imagining, from its shining Appearance, that it contained Gold. But when he had found that it did not, and had had an Opportunity, in his Tryals of admiring the Beauty of its Colour, he invented and brought into use this Preparation of it. And this is no old thing, the Invention being only of about ninety Years date; *Praxibulus* being at this Time in the Government at *Athens*.

CV. From these Accounts it is manifest, that Art imitates Nature, and sometimes produces very peculiar Things, some of which are for Use, others for Amusement only, as those employed in the ornamenting Edifices, and others, both for Amusement and Use. Such is the Production of Quicksilver [p], which has its Uses. This is obtained from

---

Vessels of a like Shape, which are buried in the Ground. After the Joinings are very firmly luted, a Fire is made about the Place, and when the Vessels grow hot, the Quicksilver gets loose, and draining through the Moss which stops the Mouth of the upper Vessel, in which it is, falls perfectly fine and pure into the lower. This is a common way at the richer Mines. At others, the Cinnabar is put into Retorts, and set in proper Furnaces, and

τριφθῇ μετ' ὄξυς ἐν ἀγγείῳ χαλκῷ, κ̀ δοίδοκι χαλκῷ. Τὰ μ̀ ἒν τοιαῦτα τάχ' ἄν τις λάβοι πλείω.

ρς'. Τῶν ἢ μεταλλευτῶν τὰ ἐν τοῖς γεωφανέσιν ἔτι λοιπά· περὶ ὧν ἡ ηὑρεσις, ὥσπερ ἐλέχθη, κατ' ἀρχὰς ἐκ ζυρρόης τινὸς κ̀ ἐκκρίσεως γίνἐ), κα-

---

and the Quickſilver is raiſed by the Heat in Fumes and falls into the Receiver, which is filled three parts with cold Water, to make it condenſe again the more readily. But there is ſome Cinnabar which contains ſo much Sulphur, that the Quickſilver it holds can never be got looſe, without the Addition of ſomething to abſorb the Sulphur. This Kind is generally deſtilled by the Retort, with Quicklime, Filings of Iron, Wood-aſhes, Salt of Tartar, Potaſhes, or ſomething of that kind. And from the Reſiduum of theſe Deſtillations, a pure and genuine *Lac Sulphuris* may be prepared, by the common way of boiling and precipitating with deſtilled Vinegar. Our factitious Cinnabar, made only by ſubliming Mercury and Sulphur together, exactly reſembles the native of ſome kinds in all its Qualities, and yields its Quickſilver pure and fluid again by the ſame Means.

But beſide all theſe ways of procuring Quickſilver from the Cinnabars, it is ſometimes found pure, unmixed, and fluid in the Bowels of the Earth. And this Kind *Dioſcorides* diſtinguiſhes by the Name of ὑδράργυρος καθ' ἑαυτόν. This is cleared from its Earth by waſhing in common Water, and from ſome other heterogene Matters, by Salt and Vinegar, and then is ſtrained through Leather, and called Virgin Quickſilver.

It is a Mineral of a perfectly ſingular kind, and when pure and unmixed, keeps conſtantly its fluid Form. It may be amalgamed with all other metallick Subſtances, but is moſt difficultly made to mix with Antimony, Iron, and Copper. It penetrates the Subſtance of all Metals, and diſſolves, and makes them brittle. It is the heavieſt of the

native Cinnabar, rubbed with Vinegar in a brass Mortar with a brass Pestle. And many other Things of this kind others, perhaps, may hit upon

CVI. There yet remain also of the fossile Kingdom certain remarkable Earths dug out of Pits, the Formation [q] of which, as was observed in the beginning of this Treatise (owing either to the mere Afflux or Percolation of their constituent Parts) is

---

Metals except Gold, which is to it as 4 to 3, or thereabout, and therefore will not swim in it, as all other Metals do. It is, however, notwithstanding its Weight, extremely volatile, and easily raised in form of a very subtle Vapour, and in that Form, dissipated entirely by means of Fire.

Quicksilver, from its ill Effects on the Miners and People employed about large Quantities of it, was long esteemed a Poison among the Antients. *Dioscorides* reckons it a thing which must have very pernicious Effects in Medicine, and *Galen* believed it highly corrosive. It first got into Use externally among the *Arabians*, and afterwards, but not till long afterwards, got introduced into the Number of internal Medicines, from the repeated Observations of its Safety and good Effects when given to Cattle, and from the hardy Attempts of some unhappy People, who had ventured to take it down in large Quantities (in order to procure Abortion) without any ill Effect

[q] The various Operations of Nature, in the Formation of these and other fossile Substances, have been treated of at large in the beginning of this Work, the greatest of all Distinctions among these, is that of such as are found in the perpendicular Fissures, and such as are deposited in Strata. The Difference between these Kinds in their degree of Purity and Fineness, is extremely great, as I have before observed, and must necessarily be so, from their different manner of Formation, as those of the perpendicular Fissures have been formed by Percolation, at different Times, and those of Strata, by mere Subsidence from among the Waters of the general Deluge.

θαρωτέρας ᾗ ὁμαλωτέρας τ̃ ἄλλων. χρώματα δὲ παντοῖα λαμβάνουσιν ᾗ διὰ τὴν τ̃ ὑποκειμένων [r] τε ᾗ διὰ τὴν τ̃ ποιούντων διαφοράν. ἐξ ὧν τὰς μελαινῶντες, τὰς δὲ τήκοντες καὶ τρίβοντες, ζωγράφεσσι τὰς λίθες τὰς ἐκ τ̃ Ἀσίας εἰς ταύτας ἀγομένας.

ρζ΄. Αἱ ὴ αὐτοφυεῖς, καὶ ἅμμα τῷ πηκτῷ τὸ χρήσιμον ἔχουσαι, σχεδὸν τρεῖς εἰσιν, ἢ τέτταρες· ἥ τε Μηλιὰς, ᾗ ἡ Κιμωλία, ᾗ ἡ Σαμία, καὶ ἡ Τυμφαϊκὴ τετάρτη παρὰ ταύτας, ἡ Γύψος.

---

[r] The high-colour'd Earths used by Painters and in Medicine, owe their several Colours, in a great measure, to the same Cause as the Gems, &c. do theirs, a Mixture of metalline Matter of various Kinds, which stains them, as it does those, with the Colour it naturally yields, in the particular kind of Solution its Particles have met with. Thus Copper, dissolved in a proper Alkali, makes, with a proper gemmeous Matter, a blue Sapphire, and with Earth, the *Lapis Armenus*, a Substance before described. And the same Particles dissolved in a proper Acid, give to gemmeous Matter the Colour which makes it an Emerald; and to Earth, that which makes it the *Terre verte*, an Earth used by our Painters, of a dusky greenish Colour, and dense, unctuous, clayey Constitution; generally brought from *Italy*, but to be met with entirely as good here at home. And Iron, which gives that glorious Red to the Ruby, the Garnet, and the Amethyst, with Earth, makes the red Boles, Ochres, and Clays.

[s] The *Melian* Earth of the Antients was a fine white Marle, of a loose crumbling Texture, and easily diffusible in Water or other Liquors. Some have imagined it to have been of other Colours, but that it was really white, we have the unquestionable Authority of the Antients *Pliny* not only describes it to be so, in his general Account of it,

from a more pure and equal Matter than the other more common Kinds. And thefe receive their various Colours from the Differences as well of their Properties of acting on other Bodies [r], as of their being subject to be acted on by them. Some of thefe they foften, and others melt, and afterwards reduce to Powder, and from thefe compofe the ftony Maffes which we receive from *Afia*.

CVII But the native, which have their Ufe as well as Excellence, are only three or four, the [s] *Melian*, the [t] *Cimolian*, the *Samian*, and the *Tymphaican*, called *Gypfum*.

---

but afterwards confirms it in another Chapter, where he fays it was the White of the great Painters of Antiquity: *Lib.* 35. *c.* 6. fpeaking of it among the other Earths, he fays, *Melinum candidum et ipfum, eft optimum in Melo infula.* And *lib.* 35 *c* 7. fpeaking of the Painters of Antiquity, he fays, *Quatuor coloribus folis, immortalia illa opera fecere, ex albis Melino, ex Silaciis Attico, ex rubris Sinopide Pontica, ex nigris Atramento.* I mention thefe two Paffages as the beft way of judging certainly from *Pliny*; for he often errs, and where he has occafion to mention the fame Subftance a fecond time, frequently contradicts what he had before faid of it. This is to be obferved in too many Places in that Author, and has arifen from this, that he was a general Collector, and often carelefly put down what different Authors had faid of the fame Subftance, either under the fame, or under different Names, in different Places of his Work, where two fuch Authors had been both uncertain as to the Truth, and probably the World in general alfo, they frequently made different Conjectures, and where one had erred, the other frequently corrected him. The Accounts of both, therefore, given by a third Perfon in their own Words, in different Parts of *Pliny*'s Hiftory, and that without mentioning them as the Opinions of different Perfons, has been the Occafion of great part of the Contradictions in that Author. But

ρή. Χρῶν] ὴ οἱ γραφεῖς τῇ Μηλιάδι μόνον, τῇ
Σαμίᾳ δ᾽ ὒ, καίπερ ὔση καλῇ, διὰ τὸ λίπος ἔχειν

where he has mentioned the same thing in different Places, and that with the same Description, I always judge he may be absolutely depended on, and that the general Opinion of the World was on his Side.

With this Account of the *Melian* Earth, as white, it is very surprising that the generality of Authors, and even those of the first Class, have constantly imagined it to be yellow. The Occasion of the Mistake has been, that the *Melinus Color* of the *Latins*, Μήλινον χρῶμα of the *Greeks*, is yellow. This, they took it for granted, had its Origin from the Colour of the *Melian* Earth, a Substance anticntly used in Painting, and which therefore they concluded must be yellow, and described it accordingly. In this manner have numberless other Errors crept into Natural History by Accident, by Mistakes in other Matters; and been afterwards sacredly propagated by a servile Sett of Writers, who have never dared to think for themselves, but have taken upon trust whatever they have found in their Ancestors Works, however dissonant to Reason, and, in many Cases, even to the Testimony of their Senses. The Occasion of this so general Error, is no more than the mistaking the Etymology of the Word Μήλινος, *Melinus*, which is not derived from Μηλιάς, or Μηλία γῆ, the *Melian* Earth here described, but from μῆλις, *pomum*, an Apple, and exactly meant that kind of yellow common on ripe Apples of many Kinds, and the strict Sense of the Verb μηλίζειν, is, according to the most correct Lexicographers, *Colore luteo esse, sive pomum referente*. These are their very Words. And hence, from an Error in a Subject foreign to Natural History, has happened, we see, an egregious Error in that Study, and which has been propagated on from Author to Author, for want of consulting even a good Lexicon.

The *Cimolian* Earth had (like the other Kinds) its Name from the Place where it was originally dug, the Island *Cimolus*. Many Authors have ranked this among the Clays, and *Tournefort* makes it a Chalk, but it appears

CVIII. Of thefe the Painters ufe only the *Melian*; they meddle not with the *Samian*, though it

to me to have been neither of thefe, but properly and diftinctly a Marle, an Earth of a middle Nature, between both. It was white, denfe, of a loofe Texture, and generally impure, having Sand or fmall Pebbles among it, infipid to the Tafte, but foft and unctuous to the Touch. Many have imagined our Fullers-earth to be the *Cimolia* of the Antients, but erroneoufly. The Subftance which comes neareft it of all the now known Foffils, is the *Steatites* of the Soap Rock of *Cornwall*, which is the common Matter of a great part of the Cliff near the *Lizard* Point. The Antients ufed their Cimola for cleaning their Cloaths. And partly from the fimilar Ufe of our Fullers-earth, and partly from an erroneous Opinion of its being the fame with that of the Antients, it has obtained the fame Name. We, indeed, know at prefent two different Subftances under this Name, with the different Epithets of *alba* and *purpurafcens*, a much more appofite one than the laft of which might eafily have been ufed. By the *Cimolia Alba*, we mean the Earth ufed for making Tobacco-pipes, and by the *Cimolia Purpurafcens*, the common Fullers-earth, of fuch conftant and important Ufe in the cleaning our woollen Cloaths.

The *Samian* Earth is a denfe, ponderous, unctuous Clay, of a fubaftringent Tafte, and either white, or afh-colour'd; it is ufed principally in Medicine, and it has the fame Virtues with the *Terra Lemnia*, and others of this Clafs, and is dug in the Ifland of *Samos*, from whence it has its Name, and never was dug in any other Place that we know of. *Pliny*, indeed, fays that it was alfo dug in the Ifland of *Melos*, but not ufed by the Painters becaufe of its Fatnefs. He errs, however, in this, which is apparently only a carelefs Tranflation of the Paffage before us. And it may be obferved, from a thoufand Inftances of this kind, how neceffary it was to bring the genuine Work of this Author on this Subject to a more frequent and eafy Ufe, to avoid the being mifled by *Pliny* and others, who have mifreprefented fo many Things from him, and given thofe Mifreprefentations and Errors, as Accounts from their own Knowledge: The

κ̀ πυκνότητα & λειότητα. τὸ γὰ ἀραιὸν ἥμερον, κỳ
τραχῶδες κỳ ἀλιπὲς, ἐπὶ τῆς γραφῆς ἁρμόζει
μᾶλλον. ὅπερ ἡ Μηλιὰς ἔχει ἐν τῷ Φάρει· εἰσὶ
κỳ ἐν τῇ Μήλῳ, κỳ ἐν τῇ Σάμῳ διαφοραὶ τῆς γῆς
πλείες.

ρθ´. Ὀρύτοντα μ̀ ἓν ὀυκ ἔςιν ὀρθὸν ςῆσαιᵛ ἐν τοῖς
ἐν Σάμῳ, ἀλλ᾽ ἀναγκαῖον ἢ ὕπτιον, ἢ πλάγιον. ἡ
δ᾽ φλὲψ ἐπὶ πολὺ διατείνει· τὸ μ̀ ὕψῷ ἡλίκη

Paſſage in *Pliny* is, *Melinum candidum et ipſum eſt optimum in Milo inſula, in Samo naſcitur, ſed eo non viuntur Pictores propter pinguitudinem.* It is moſt evident, that this is taken from the Paſſage now before us in *Theophraſtus*, but *Pliny* deviates from his Original into a very great Error in it *Theophraſtus* does not ſay, that the *Melian* Earth was dug in *Samos*, and was not uſed by the Painters, but that the *Samian* Earth, another Subſtance which he had juſt before mentioned, and was about to ſay ſomething more about, was not uſed by them, and adds, that in both theſe Places there were many various Kinds of Earth, but not that the Kind named from either, was found in the other

ᵛ Our Author's Account of this Earth, and the manner of digging it, has been generally copied by thoſe who have deſcribed it ſince *Pliny* ſays, *accubantes effodiunt ibi inter ſaxa venas ſcrutantes* And in another Place, *Samiæ duæ ſunt, quæ Syropicon* (or *Collyrion*) *et quæ Aſter appellantur* And other of the old Authors much to the ſame Effect.

I have before obſerved, that this Earth was either white or aſh-colour'd, theſe two Colours conſtituted the Difference between the two Kinds, and were what were called the *Aſter* and *Collyrion* The white was the *Aſter*, ſuppoſed by many to be a Talc, and ſo called, for its ſhining, and the aſh-coloured was called, from its Colour, *Collyrion*,

is very beautiful, becaufe it is fat, denfe, and unctuous; whereas fuch as are of a loofer Texture,
crumbling, dry, and without Fatnefs, are fitter
for their Ufe, all which Properties the *Melian*,
particularly that of *Pharis*, poffeffes. There are,
however, befide thefe, in *Melos* and *Samos* both,
many various kinds of Earths.

CIX The Diggers in the Pits of *Samos* cannot
ftand upright ʷ at their Work, but are forced to lie
along, either on their Backs or on one Side; for
the Vein of the Earth they dig runs length-way,
and is only of the depth of about two Foot, tho'

Κλλύςον Κολλύρα among the *Greeks* fignified a kind of
Loaf baked in Afhes, and commonly brought to the Colour of the Afhes in the doing. And from a Refemblance
to this was this Earth called *Collyrion*, or the afh-colour'd
Samian Earth.

Pliny imagined it had this Name from its being a common Ingredient in certain Medicines for the Eyes, commonly
called *Collyria*, but *Dioscorides*, from whom he took the
occafion of this Conjecture, does not attribute this Quality
to the *Samian* Earth of either kind, but to the *Lapis Sa-
mius*, a Stone found among it. And from this Error alone
it is, that fo many have imagined that the *Samian* Earth
was ufed in Medicines for the Eyes. Indeed when an
Error in regard to the Antients is once fet on foot, there
is no knowing what a Series of different Miftakes may be
the Confequences of it. Thefe Medicines for the Eyes,
called *Collyria*, though they did not give the Name to the
afh-colour'd *Samian* Earth fo called, may ferve, however,
to confirm the Opinion of its having it on occafion of its
Colour refembling that of Afhes, fince they had theirs
from the fame Caufe, and were only called *Collyria*, that
is afh-colour'd Medicines, from their being made of Subftances of the Tutty kind, and refembling Afhes in Colour.

L 2

δίπυς, τὸ δὲ βάθ@ πολλῷ μεῖζον· ἐφ' ἑκάτερα δ' αὐτῶ λίθοι περιέχυσιν ἐξ ὧν ἐξαιρεῖται. Διαφυὴν ἔχει διὰ μέσε, ἡ ἡ Διαφυὴ βελτίων ἐστὶ τῆς ἔξω. ἡ πάλιν ἑτέραν αὐτῆς καὶ ἑτέραν ἄχρι τεττάρων ἐστίν, ἔχυσα ἡ ἐσχάτη καλεῖται Ἀστήρ.

ρι. Χρῶν] δὲ τῇ γῇ πρὸς τὰ ἱμάτια, μάλιστα Κιμωλίᾳ. Χρῶν] δὲ τῇ Τυμφαϊκῇ πρὸς τὰ ἱμάτια, ἡ καλῦσι ʷ Γύψον, οἱ περὶ Τυμφαίαν ἡ τὰς τόπυς ἐκείνυς.

ʷ The Antients had many kinds of *Gypsum*, very different from one another, and used for different Purposes. but the principal Kinds were three, 1. the *Terra Tymphaica Gypsum incolis dicta*, Γῆ Τυμφαϊκή ἣν οἱ περὶ Τυμφαίαν ἡ τὰς τόπυς, ἐκεῖ ἃς καλῦσι Γύψον, The *Tymphaican* Earth, called by the Inhabitants *Gypsum*, 2. the real genuine *Gypsum*, which was made, by burning, from a certain talcy Substance of the *Lapis Specularis* kind; and 3 that made by burning many different Species of Stones of the Alabaster and other similar kinds.

The *Tymphaican* here mentioned appears to have been an Earth approaching to the nature of the Marles, but with this remarkable Quality, that it would make a kind of Plaister or Cement by mixing with Water, without having passed the Fire. This Substance is yet to be found in many Places carefully sought after. I remember to have taken up an Earth, which I found to have this Property, near *Goodwood*, the Seat of his Grace the Duke of *Richmond*, in *Sussex*. And Mr. *Morton* is recorded to have sent to Dr. *Woodward*, from *Clipston* Stone-pit in *Northamptonshire*, an Earth truly of this kind, and endued with this Quality, under the Name of *Calx Nativa*. His is described to be a whitish gritty Earth, but what I found was a true genuine Marle, something loose in Texture, but with no Sand or other stony

2

much more in breadth, and is inclosed in on every side with Stones, from between which it is taken. There is also in the Mass of the Vein a distinct Stratum near the middle, which is of better Earth than that without it, and within that there is sometimes another yet finer; and even beyond that a fourth. The fartheft of these is that which is called the *After*.

CX. Earths of some kinds are also used about Cloaths, particularly the *Cimolian* The *Tymphaican* is also used for the same Purposes, and the People of *Tymphæa* and the neighbouring Places call it *Gypsum*.

Matter among it, and of this kind the *Gypsum Tymphaicum* evidently was. This Author calls it an Earth only, and observes, that the People about the Places where it was found called it *Gypsum*, I suppose from its having the Properties of that Substance. As to its Use about Cloaths, the Substance I picked up in *Sussex* seemed of a Texture so much resembling that of Fullers-earth, that if it could be conveniently used, it seemed to promise to answer all the Purposes of it, and so did the *Gypsum Tymphaicum* of the Antients, of which *Pliny* expressly says, *Græcia pro Cimolia Tymphaico utitur Gypso*, lib. 36. c. 17.

This therefore, or something like this, must be the first of the three principal *Gypsums* of the Antients, the other two Kinds I shall have occasion to mention hereafter, but must first observe, in regard to this Passage, that it has been strangely corrupted in different Copies; instead of Τύλα, it is in several ἴχον, and what I have given Κιμωλία, from the very judicious Conjecture of *De Laet*, is in most Copies ἡ μόνον. The Use of our Fullers-earth about Cloaths, and, in all probability, that of the *Cimolia* of the Antients, was the same, this is not only that trifling one, of the taking out accidental Spots of Grease got in the wearing, but what is the most important of all things in the Woollen Cloth Manufacture, the cleansing the Pieces of it, at the

ριά. Ἡ ὃ Γύψ@ γίν) πλείςη μ͂ ἐν Κύπρῳˣ, ᷓ πεϊφανεϛάτη. μικρὸν ϒ̄ ἀφαιρϖσι τ͂ γῆς ὀρύτ-
τον]ες. ἐν Φοινίκη ϳ καὶ ἐν ʸ Συρίᾳ καίον]ες τὰς

---

time of making, from that vast Quantity of Greafe, Tar, and other Filth they are fouled with, from the Tar and Greafe ufed externally in the Diforders of the Sheep before fhorn, and the Oil neceffary to be thrown into the Cloath in the working.

ˣ The *Cyprian Gypfum* here mentioned I account a different kind from the *Tymphaan*, and to be, indeed, the true genuine *Gypfum* made from the talcy Subftance before mentioned. *Pliny* feems to favour this Divifion of the *Gypfums* into three Kinds, where he fays, lib. 36. c. 23. *Cognita Calcireis Gypfum eft, plura ejus genera. Nam e Lapide coquitur, ut in Syria et Thuriis & e terra foditur, ut in Cypro & Perilibus, e fumma tellure & Tymphaicum eft.* And according to this, the three Kinds before diftinguifhed may be called the *Tymphæan, Cyprian,* and *Syrian*. The *Tymphæan* is the earthy one already defcribed, which might, very probably, be found near the Surface, as being truly an Earth, not a Stone. The fecond is the true genuine *Gypfum*, made from the Talc, or *Lapis Specularis*, called alfo, for that Reafon, *Metallum Gypfinum*. And the third, the Kind made from the Alabafters and other Stones of a fimilar Texture.

That this *Cyprian Gypfum*, or that Kind burnt from the *Lapis Specularis*, or genuine *Metallum Gypfinum*, was the fineft and beft of all the Kinds, we have alfo *Pliny*'s Word, lib 36. c. 24. *Omnium autem optimum fieri compertum eft e lapide fpeculari fquamamve talem habente.*

ʸ The *Syrian*, or third kind of *Gypfum*, this Author here obferves, was made by burning certain Stones, which he afterwards very well defcribes, and which we may fee from his Account were of the very Kind with thofe we now principally ufe for that Purpofe, and call *Parget*, or Plaifter-ftone, different kinds of which are dug in *Derbyfhire*

CXI. *Gypsum* is produced in great Quantities in the Island of *Cyprus*[x], where it lies open, and easy to be discovered, and come at, the Workmen having but very little Earth to take away before they get it. In *Phœnicia* and *Syria* also they have a

---

and *Yorkshire* in *England*, and the Pits of *Montmartre* in *France*. There are many other Kinds in different Parts, both of *France* and *England*, very little different from these and from each other; but in general all of them very well answer the Description *Theophrastus* gives of the Stones from which what I have called the *Syrian Gypsum* of the Antients was made.

It is to be observed that we, as well as the Antients, burn many very different Stones into our *Gypsum*, or Plaister of Paris, as it is commonly called; some of which are of the Nature of the foliaceous, others of the fibrous Talcs, others composed of Matter seeming the same with that of the Talcs, but amassed together in a different Form, being neither fibrous nor foliaceous, but seemingly in coarse Powder or arenaceous Particles of uncertain Figures, and held together in the same manner as the Grit of the Stone of Strata. And others truly and legitimately of the Alabaster kind; in many of these, Particles of genuine sparry Matter also discover themselves, and in several, the Masses are wholly surrounded with, and in many Places their very Substance penetrated by a reddish earthy Matter. These require different degrees of burning, according to their different Texture, to bring them to the State proper for use. But in most of them it is done in a very little time, and by a very slight Calcination, in comparison to that required for equally altering most other Substances. And the reddish Kinds burn to a Gypsum, equally white with that made from the whitest. The Gypsum of *Montmartre* in *France*, the best and finest in the World, is burnt to a proper State in about two Hours. Ours of *Derbyshire* takes but little more time if properly managed, and that of *Yorkshire*, which is generally redder and coarser, a little more than that. We have no Opportunities of try-

(152)

λίθες ποιᾶσιν. ἔπειτα δ' ἐν Θυρέοις. ἢ γδ ἐκεῖ γίνε] πολλή. τρίτη δ' ἡ περὶ Τυμφαίαν, ἢ περὶ Περαιβίαν, ἢ κατ' ἄλλες τόπες. ἡ ῥ φύσις αὐτῶν ἰδία. λιθωδεςτέρα γδ μᾶλλόν ἐςιν ἢ γεώδης.

ριβ'. Ὁ ἢ λίθος ἐμφερὴς τῷ ᾿Αλαβαςρίτῃ. μέγας δ' ἐ τέμνε], ἀλλὰ χαλικώδης. ἡ ῥ γλιχρότης ἢ θερμότης, ὅταν βρεχθῇ, θαυμαςή.

...ing the *Lapis Specularis* of the Antients now, but by the general Consent of the Writers of Antiquity, the *Gypsum* made of it exceeded all the other Kinds, the Substance itself from this obtained a Name by which it became afterwards generally known, which was *Gypsinum metallum*. The want of knowing this, however, among the Commentators on some of the Works of the Writers since, has occasioned much blundering, for finding Accounts, in the most express Words, of Windows and Reflecting Mirrors, made of the *Metallum Gypsum*, and not conceiving that this was only another Name for the *Lapis Specularis*, which it had obtained from being the Matter of which *Gypsum* was made, they made no scruple of blotting out the Word *Gypsinum*, because they did not understand it, a Thing too customary among this Sett of People, and supplied its place with *Gypsinum*, leaving a Passage which they imagined very dark, much darker than they found it.

[z] *Pliny says*, the Stones burnt to make *Gypsum* ought to be of the Marble or Alabaster kind, and that in *Syria* they chuse the hardest they can get. Lib 36 c 24. *Qui coquitur Lapis non aliter debet esse dilectu ac marmoroso, in Syria duritia saligna etc*. His Commentators say he took this from this Author, *hæc ex Theophrasti*, lib. *περὶ λίθε, De*. It he did, he has been very careless in his translating him, a Fault I have been obliged to observe in some other Places, that he is too apt to be guilty of. In

Gypsum, which they make by burning certain Stones. They have a *Gypsum* in *Thuria* too, in great plenty; as also about *Tymphæa*, and in the Country of the *Perrhæbeans*, and many other Places; but these are of a peculiar Kind, and are rather of a stony, than of an earthy Texture.

CXII. The Stone from which *Gypsum* is made, by burning, is like ͫ Alabaster; it is not dug, however, in such large Masses, but in separate Lumps. Its Viscidity and Heat, when moistened, are very wonderful.

---

this Passage, however, I am of opinion he is not justly to be accused of it; for, with his Commentators Leave, I must observe, that it appears very plainly, from this and the Context, that he did not take this from *Theophrastus*. This Author does not say, that they chose in *Syria* the hardest Stones, but τὰς ἁπλουστέρας, those of the simplest Texture; and the Remainder of the Sentence in *Pliny*, which is, *coquuntque fimo bubulo ut celerius uriantur*, being evidently from some other Source, as there is not the least Syllable of any thing like it in this Author, makes it probable, that he had it together from some other Writer, or from the common Tradition of his Time. I must confess, the Word ςερεωτάτους coming so close after the μαρμάρους κỳ ἁπλουστέρους, would have made me very naturally suspect *Pliny* of taking his Account carelessly from this Author, but the Context, which is evidently not hence, may very reasonably clear him. This I have been the more particular in observing here, as it may be a Means of clearing that Author in some, at least, of the many Passages in which he may be even more than he deserves accused of misunderstanding the Authors he copied from, in too many Places he has indeed but too evidently done this, though in some, where he is suspected of it, perhaps he may not be copying from the Authors we accuse him of misrepresenting, but from others, who had either accidentally, or purposely, deviated from what those had written, and whose Works may be now lost to us.

(154)

ριγ΄. Χρῶνται γὰ πρός τε τὰ οἰκοδομήματα τούτου τοῦ λίθου περιέχοντες. κἄν τε ἄλλο βέλωνται τούτο κολλῆσαι. κόψαντες ϡ, κὴ ὕδωρ ἐπιχέοντες, ταράτ]ωσι ξύλοις. τῇ χειρὶ γὰ οὐ δύνανται, διὰ τὴν θερμότητα. βρέχουσι ϡ παραχρῆμα πρὸς τὴν χρείαν, ἐὰν μικρὸν πρότερον ταχὺ πήγνυται· κὴ οὐκ ἔςι διελθεῖν ἅμα.

ριδ΄. Ἔςι ϡ κὴ ἰσχυς. ὅτε γὰ οἱ τοῖχοι ῥήγνυνται κὴ διαφθείρονται, ἡ δ' ἄμμος ἀνίησι. πολλάκις ϡ ὃ τὰ μ̄ πέπ]ωκε κὴ ὑφήρη]. τὰ δ' ἄνω κρεμάμλυα κὴ ζυνεχόμλυα τῇ κολλήσ૬.

ριέ. Δύναται ϡ κὴ ὑφαιρεμλύη, πάλιν κὴ πάλιν ὀπ]ᾶσθ, ὃ γίνεσθ χρησίμη. Περὶ μ̄ οὖν Κύπρον κὴ Φοινίκην εἰς ταῦτα μάλιςα. περὶ δ' Ἰταλίαν κὴ εἰς τὴν ᵃ κονίασιν ὃ οἱ γραφεῖς ἔνια τ κατ τὴν τέχνην. ἔτι ϡ οἱ κναφεῖς ἐμπάτ]οντες εἰς τὰ ἱμάτια.

ᵃ What I have given εἰς τὴν κονίασιν, speaking of the Use of the Gypsum in Italy, has stood in most Copies εἰς τὴν οἰκίαν, which has been distrusted by many not to be the genuine Reading but imagined by *Furlan* to have been

CXIII They use this in Buildings, casing them with it, or putting it on any particular Place they would strengthen. They prepare it for Use, by reducing it to Powder, and then pouring Water on it, and stirring and mixing the Matter well together with wooden Instruments: For they cannot do this with the Hand because of the Heat. They prepare it in this manner immediately before the Time of using it, for in a very little while after moistening, it dries and becomes hard, and not in a Condition to be used.

CXIV. This Cement is very strong, and often remains good, even after the Walls it is laid on crack and decay, and the Sand of the Stone they are built with moulders away; for it is often seen, that even after some part of a Wall has separated itself from the rest, and is fallen down, other parts of it shall yet hang together, and continue firm and in their Place, by means of the Strength of this Matter which they are covered with.

CXV This *Gypsum* may also be taken off from Buildings, and by burning, again and again, be made fit for Use. It is used for the casing the Outsides of Edifices, principally in *Cyprus* and *Phœnicia*, but in *Italy*, for [a] whitening over the Walls, and other kind of Ornaments within Houses. Some Kinds of it are also used by Painters in their Business, and by the Fullers, about Cloaths.

---

erroneously put for τις τὸ ὄνον, and he has translated the Passage accordingly, the ν ιλασιν is from the Opinion of *Salmasius*, and seems to have been the very Meaning of the Author, for having been just before mentioning its Use on

ριϛ'. Διαφέρειν ἢ δοκεῖ καὶ πρὸς τὰ ἀπομάγματα πολὺ τῶν ἄλλων. Εἰς ὃ καὶ χρῶνἸ μᾶλλον, καὶ μάλιϑ' οἱ περὶ τὴν Ἑλλάδα, γλισχρότητι καὶ λειότητι.

ριζ'. Ἡ μὲν δύναμις ἐν τούτοις καὶ τοῖς πιϛτοῖς. ἡ δὲ φύσις ἔοικεν ἀμφότερά πως ἔχειν, καὶ κατὰ τὰ τῆς κονίας, καὶ κατὰ τὰ τῆς γῆς, θερμότητα καὶ γλισχρότητα. μᾶλλον δὲ ἑκατέρας ὑπερεχούσας. θερμοτέρα γὰρ τῆς κονίας, γλισχροτέρα δὲ πολὺ τῆς γῆς.

ριη'. Ὅτι δ' ἔμπυρος, κἀκεῖθεν φανερόν. ἤδε γάρ τις ναῦς ἱματηγὸς, βρεχθέντων ἱματίων, ὡς ἐμπυρώθησαν, ζυγκατεκαύθη καὶ αὐτή.

ριθ'. Καίουσι δὲ καὶ ἐν Φοινίκῃ, καὶ ἐν Συρίᾳ, καμινδ'οντες αὐτὴν καὶ καίοντες. καίουσι δὲ μάλιϛα τοὺς μαρμάρους καὶ ἀπλουϛέρους· ϛερεοτάτους μὲν προτιθέντες διὰ τὸ θᾶττον καίεϛϑαι καὶ μᾶλλον. δοκεῖ γὰρ θερμότατον εἶναι πυρωθέν, καὶ πλεῖϛον χρόνον διαρκεῖ. ὀπτήσαντες δὲ κόπτουσιν ὥσπερ τὴν κονίαν.

---

the Outsides of Houses, and being going on to recount its other various Uses, there was nothing so natural for him to

CXVI. It is also excellent, and superior to all other Things, for making Images; for which it is greatly used, and especially in *Greece*, because of its Pliableness and Smoothness.

CXVII. These Qualities of the *Gypsum*, therefore, fit it for these and such other Uses, for it seems naturally to have, as it were together, the Heat, and Tenacity of Lime, and the more viscous Earths. But it possesses both these Qualities in a much superior degree to either of the others, which have them singly; for it acquires, on being moistened, a Heat much greater than that of Lime, and is much more tenacious than the most viscous of the Earths.

CXVIII. That its fiery Power is very great, is evident from this remarkable Instance. That a certain Ship which was laden with Cloaths, by some Accident letting in Water, the Cloaths being wetted by that means, the *Gypsum* that was put among them took fire, and burnt both the Cloaths and the Ship.

CXIX. In *Syria* and *Phœnicia* they prepare a *Gypsum* by Fire; putting into proper Furnaces Stones, principally of the Marble, and other Kinds, which are of the most simple Texture, and heating them to a certain degree, the harder Kinds they lay upon those which burn more readily, and when burnt, the Matter appears to be of extreme Strength, and fitted for enduring a long time. After this they beat the Stones to powder like Lime, to make them fit for Use.

---

mention next, as its Use in ornamenting the inner parts of them, the very thing it is most famous for now.

ρκ. Ἐκ τύτυ δ' ἂν δόξειεν εἶναι φανερὸν ὅτι πυρώδης τις ἡ γένεσις αὐτὴ τὸ ὅλον ἐςίν [b].

---

[b] The Obſervation the Author concludes this Work with is unqueſtionably moſt juſt. We are well acquainted with the many Changes which the Particles of Fire, inſinuating themſelves into Bodies, are able to make, of which, their

FINIS.

CXX. From all this it seems evident, that the Properties and Nature of this Matter, are in a great degree owing to the Fire [b].

---

changing the Talcs and Alabasters into *Gypsum*, and the Lime-stones of various kinds into Lime, are not the least worthy our Observation, though from their being common and every day before our Eyes, they are but little regarded.

F I N I S.

TWO LETTERS:

ONE, TO

Dr. JAMES PARSONS, F.R.S.

On the Colours of the SAPPHIRE and TURQUOISE.

Read before the ROYAL SOCIETY, Thursday, June 19, 1746.

AND THE OTHER,

To MARTIN FOLKES, *Esq*;

DOCTOR of LAWS, and PRESIDENT of the ROYAL SOCIETY.

On the Effects of different Menstruums on COPPER.

LETTER I.

TO

Dr. JAMES PARSONS, F.R.S.

On the Colours of the SAPPHIRE and TURQUOISE.

Read before the ROYAL SOCIETY, Thursday, June 19, 1746.

SIR,

WHEN the Specimen I have ventured to publish of my Notes on THEOPRHASTUS was favourably mentioned Yesterday, by you and some other Gentlemen, whose good Opinions I am very sensible how much Reason I have to be proud of; you may remember that some of the Company objected to the *Sapphire*'s being coloured by Particles of *Copper*, and seemed very firm in the Opinion, that that Gem owes its Colour to a *Native Zaffer*.

I am sorry I have only Room to name Things in those Notes, without Opportunities of entering into a Detail of the Experiments by which I have generally been able to give convincing Proofs of the Truth of I what assert. Had I Room there to give an Account, as I could wish, of these, or enter at large into the Arguments founded on them, I am apt to believe many Objections of this kind would have been obviated. But as it has been impossible for me to do this every where in the course of that Work, it may not be improper to take this Opportunity of entering more at large into the Reasons which have induced me to be of the Opinion that has given Rise to this Objection, and endeavour, by Arguments founded only on Facts, and a strict and impartial Observation of Nature, to settle the great Question among the more eminent of the later Naturalists, Whether it be to a *Native Zaffer*, or to Particles of *Copper*, that the blue Gems in general owe their Colour.

I need not tell You, who are so well acquainted with the Works of the *French* Naturalists, that the *Sapphires* being coloured by a *Native Zaffer*, is not the Opinion of those Gentlemen alone who now made the Objection, but many have favoured it, and it is at present generally received.

For my own Part, you will observe, through the Course of those Notes, that I have not tied myself down to the Sentiments of any particular Author, but have, as my own Experiments and Observations directed, at Times agreed to, and in other Places disputed, the Opinions of the whole Number, both of

Philosophers and Critics, and as Experiments, the only sure Guides to Knowledge, have led me to it, have adopted, or dissented from their Opinions. How I have succeeded in this in the Example before us, the fairest way of judging will be first, fairly to give the Arguments used in Support of the other, and common Opinion, which are principally three, and which have the Appearance of being of some Weight. They are.

1. That the *Turquoise* is evidently coloured by the same Matter with the *Sapphire*, and that the Matter of its Colour is known to be a *Native Zaffer*.

2. That *Copper* is not capable of giving the deep Blue of some of the deeper *Sapphires*, and *Veins* and *Striæ* of the rough native *Turquoises*

3. That *Zaffer* is the Substance which colours the common blue Glass, and that it is capable of giving the Colour of the deepest native *Sapphires*; as is evident from the counterfeit ones which are coloured with it, and are of all the Degrees of Colour of the genuine.

To which permit me to answer,

First, That it was incumbent on the Assertors of this Doctrine, to have proved the Existence, and examined the Nature and Properties, of this *Native Zaffer*, before they attributed such great Effects to it. I am not ashamed to say, that I don't know what *Native Zaffer* is; that I never yet saw any such Fossil, nor believe I ever shall, and notwithstanding that Dr. *Woodward*, and some other able Naturalists have ventured to name some of their unknown Specimens native *Zaffers*, I cannot bring myself to think that Nature ever formed any Substance that could be properly so called; all that I have been shewn as such, having been Things which a little Chemistry was able to shew that Naturalists ought to have been ashamed of calling by such a Name. Not that I would pretend to limit the Operations of Nature within the Bounds of our narrow Understandings, or declare any thing impossible, because it has not yet been seen to be effected, but I think the Assertors of such great Effects from so very uncertain a Substance, ought, if ever they had seen it, to have given a more rational Account of it than any we have at present.

The *Zaffer* we know, and with which the blue Glass and counterfeit *Sapphires* are stained, is a Preparation which seems to owe its present Mode of Existence merely to the extreme Force of Fire, and is perhaps no genuine Production of Nature, even in a latent State, except in its constituent Principles; but such another Substance as the lixivial Salt of Plants, which though always producible from its Subject by Fire, was not inherent in it, in that Form, (as it evidently never was, notwithstanding the erroneous Opinions of some Persons, founded on the Observation of a slight Fermentation of some parts of Vegetables with particular Acids) but produced by the extreme Force of Fire uniting the essential Salt of the Plant with its Earth and a little of its Oil. This *Zaffer* is prepared from *Cobalt*, a metallic Mineral of *Saxony*, and other Places, in some degree resembling Antimony, and affording, by the Assistance of Fire, the Arsenics, this Substance, and *Smalt*, with the Addition of a fix'd Alkali. After the Fire of a reverberatory Furnace has driven off the arsenical Particles, the remaining Mass is powdered and calcined three or four times over; and then being mixed with three times its Quantity of powdered Flints, affords us the common *Zaffer* This is the Preparation of that Body, and how likely we are ever to find a Substance truly of this Kind *native* in the Bowels of the Earth, it is easy to judge.

But as Conjectures, however rational, ought never to be made the Basis to found Arguments on in Cases of this kind, it may not be improper to examine what Weight, even allowing the Existence of a *native Zaffer*, there is in the Arguments founded on its supposed Effects

And to the *First*, That the *Turquoise* and *Sapphire* are coloured by the same Matter, and that that Matter is universally allowed to be a *native Zaffer*; I shall take the Liberty to answer, That I allow the *Sapphire* and *Turquoise* to be coloured by Particles of the same Kind; that I know it to be the common Opinion, that the *Turquoise* is coloured by *Zaffer*, and not by *Copper*, but that I also know it to be an erroneous one. I am very sensible that many Great Men, and some particularly, for whom I have in general the highest Esteem, have countenanced this Opinion, but cannot fear to dissent from them, since I am able to produce the Testimony of the Senses, that the *Turquoise* owes its Colour to *Copper* only, having succeeded in a Course of Experiments, by which I have been able to divest the *Turquoise* wholly of its Colour; to precipitate and preserve that Colour separate and alone, to prove that Colour, by the Effects of different Menstruums, to be absolute Copper, and by Experiments founded on this Process, to give, by a Solution of Copper in a volatile Alkali, the true *Turquoise* Colour to the Substance of the *native Turquoises*, which is absolutely no other than animal Bone, and make, by that means, those fictitious *Turquoises* which you have seen put, before a judicious Assembly, to the severest Tryals, and giving all the Marks of the genuine. I send you with this a Specimen of one of those very Pieces, which you will find has suffered no Change in its Colour since, and shall hereafter do myself the Honour of communicating the whole Process to the ROYAL SOCIETY.

To the *Second* Argument, That *Copper* is not capable of giving so deep a Blue as that of some of these Gems, I have to answer, That Experiments have taught me that it can; and, as a Proof of it, I send you a Specimen of a Solution of *Copper*, the very one with which I stained the factitious *Turquoises*, which you will find of the true Colour of the deepest Male *Sapphires*, and deeper than the commonly called *black Veins* of the rough native *Turquoises*, if carefully examined.

The Authors of this Objection might, indeed, have known, from the excellent Mr *Boyle*'s Experiments, that *Copper* is the last Thing to be, with any shew of Reason, suspected of wanting this Property; for that Gentleman has proved, that a Grain of that Metal is capable of giving a blue Colour to 530,620 times its Bulk of Water. And when the Arguers for the Colour of these Gems being from *Zaffer*, and not this Metal, consider in how extremely small a Quantity the metalline Particles, be they of what Kind soever, can be supposed to be mixed with the Matter of the Gems, I am apt to believe they will find this Quality so remarkable in *Copper*, and wanting in *Zaffer* a thing of the first Consequence.

In regard to the *Third* Argument, That the genuine *Sapphires* are probably coloured by *Zaffer*, because blue Glass, and the common counterfeit *Sapphires* are so; I cannot but observe, that I should as soon infer, from the *Prussian Blue*'s striking the Colour of the *Sapphire* on Canvas, that the Gem owed its Dye to *Blood*, as think an Argument of any weight could be deduced from that Observation. External Appearances are of little weight in Philosophy; and I am sorry to say, that it was only a very superficial View of these Things, that could start an Objection to *Copper*'s colouring the *Sapphire*, from them; for a more careful Examination of these very Bodies, must afford Arguments for the contrary, as it will evidently prove, that the Colour of the *Sapphire* cannot be owing to the same Substance with that of these Glasses: the very Heat necessary for forming them, would, in a few Minutes, wholly divest the finest *Sapphire* in the world of all its Colour.

Experiments of this kind are not, indeed, in every body's Way, but it is eafy to propofe one on the fame Foundation, which it is in every one's Power readily to try, and which will equally and unanfwerably prove the Truth of the Arguments founded on it.

The common blue Glafs is made from the common or cryftal *Frit* melted with *Zaffer*; and the fineft counterfeit *Sapphires*, with a cryftal *Glafs*, work'd with an Admixture of *Lead*, and this *Zaffer*, in the Proportion of about One fiftieth part. The *Lead* gives, in this Cafe, an additional Denfity to the Glafs, which adds greatly to the Luftre of the counterfeit Gem; as the more denfe the tranfparent Matter is, the more bright and vivid the metalline Tinge appears through it; but while *Lead* thus increafes the Denfity, it debafes the Glafs in another refpect of equal Confequence, in that it makes it fofter. Whichever of thefe Subftances, however, is made the Subject of this Experiment, the Effect will be the fame; for if we bring to the Tryal of only a clear Charcoal Fire, a genuine *Sapphire*, and either of thefe factitious Subftances, and throw them together into it, we fhall foon fee that they owe their Colours to Particles of a very different kind; for the Genuine will be feen to emit a fine clear blue Flame, the Counterfeit not fo much as the leaft Vapour, and when, after this, they are taken out together, the true *Sapphire* fhall be found wholly colourlefs and tranfparent, as a piece of Cryftal, and the Counterfeit or Glafs, unaltered. Thus,

and the Deadness of the one, though ever so well coloured, compared to the native vivid Brightness of the other, must evidently shew the Difference of the Substances to which those Colours are owing.

Fire, which is thus able to divest the *Sapphire* of its Colour, has also the same Effect on the *Turquoise*, as the Workers on it well know: And this is easily accounted for, if they are coloured, as I am convinced they are, by a fine metalline *Sulphur*. But I will venture to affirm, that it could not be the Case, if those Gems were coloured by a *Zaffer*.

Let it not be here objected, that the Workers on the native *Turquoises* are obliged to have Recourse to Fire to give them their Colour, and that therefore it is not probable, that the same Power should be able to take it away; for the Truth of this, is only, that the Colour of the native *Turquoises* of some Countries, is not equally spread through the whole Mass, but lodged in different Parts of it in form of *Veins* and *Siitæ*. It is to dislodge the Colour from these *Veins*, and diffuse it equally thro' the whole Mass, that they have Recourse to Heat; a very gentle Heat is all they dare trust on this Occasion, and is always found sufficient. And what I would observe from the Whole of this is, that this Effect of Fire on the rough *Turquoises*, is a Proof that their Colour is owing to the same Particles with that of the *Sapphire*; and that this dislodging and diffusing it through the whole Mass, is the first Step toward the dissipating and entirely driving it off; for a little too long Continuance in the fame Heat, will, as the Workmen too often find to their Sorrow, wholly drive off the Blue, and leave the Matter colourlefs, as the *Sapphire* when taken from the Fire.

Thus have I endeavoured to prove, in anfwer to the Arguments ufed in Support of the *Sapphire's* being coloured by a *native Zaffer* (befide the too great Probability, that there is no fuch Subftance in Nature as this *native Zaffer*) that the *Turquoife* is coloured by the fame Means with that Gem, and both by *Copper* That *Copper* is, of all Bodies in the foffile World, moft capable of diffufing its Colour; and that the blue Glafs and counterfeit *Sapphires* being coloured by *Zaffer*, are a Proof that the genuine *Sapphire* is not fo

And thus eafily are Objections of this kind anfwered, when brought to a fair Hearing; but the Misfortune is, that many of them never are fo. And permit me to add, that thefe idle Cavils ftrike at the Root of all Philofophy. The Affertors of this Opinion, perhaps, do not confider the Confequences of it If they will not allow *Copper* to colour this Gem, the fame Reafonings muft lead them to deny, that the reft of the coloured Gems owe their different Dyes to metalline Particles: And where would they propofe to find *native Zaffers* of the proper Colours for them all?

A little Obfervation indeed of Nature in her other Works of this kind, might alone have been, one would think, sufficient to have prevented such Objections as these. For why should a Man who sees that the *Vitriol*, which has *Copper* for its Basis, is blue, and knows that the *Lapis Lazuli* and *Lapis Armenus* are *Copper* Ores, that the Crystals and Spars about *Copper* Mines are very often blue, and that very many of the Ores of that Metal are of a true *Sapphire* Colour, hesitate at believing that Gem to owe its Colour to the same Metal?

I am, with all Respect,

S I R,

Broad-way, Westminster,
June 19, 1746.

Your most Obedient

Humble Servant,

JOHN HILL.

LETTER II.

TO

MARTIN FOLKES, *Esq*;

DOCTOR of LAWS; and

PRESIDENT of the ROYAL SOCIETY.

On the Effects of different Menstruums on COPPER.

SIR,

IN a Letter to Dr PARSONS of the 19*th* of the last Month, which you did me the Honour to have read before the ROYAL SOCIETY, at their meeting on the same Day, I endeavoured, principally by means of some Experiments I had been lately making, to settle the Question so much disputed among the present Naturalists, Of what the blue Gems in general are coloured from. What engaged me in the Dispute at that Time, was an Objection raised against the Opinion I had declared myself of in this Case, in the Specimen of my Notes on *Theophrastus.* And I am very happy to find, that even the Gentlemen who made that Objection are now convinced, that it is to *Copper* alone that the *Sapphire* and *Turquoise* owe their beautiful Blue,

For myself, I must acknowledge that tho' I have long been convinced of the Fact, the Manner in which it was effected, was long a great Difficulty to me: The Menstruum in which my Tincture of *Copper*, which proved to the Senses, that *Copper* was capable of giving the deepest and finest Blue imaginable, was made, was a volatile alkaline Spirit: And where Nature could find in the Bowels of the Earth any thing analogous to a volatile urinous Alkali produced by Chemistry, was a Question not easily answered. The particular Salt of the mineral Waters seems to approach, indeed, something to a Menstruum of this kind, and Dr. *Hoffman* has proved, that it is at least much fitter to be classed with the Alkalies than with the Acids. But the System of the Colours of the blue Gems being from *Copper*, must stand upon a very precarious Basis, if there could be found no other Menstruum than one we are so very uncertain about, to strike their Colour from that Metal.

Copper, however, is, in truth, perhaps the farthest of all the Metals from being subject only to the Power of one appropriated Menstruum; and a Course of Experiments on it, have now shewn me, that we need not have Recourse to so uncertain a mineral Substance as this latent Alkali, for producing a Blue from it; but that Menstruums of another kind, even Acids, and those the very Acids, whose Principles are the commonest of all others in the Earth, can afford us the same Colour from it, and are every where to be found in great abundance.

Gold is foluble only in *Aqua regia*, for all the other Menftruums that are talk'd of for it, have a genuine Sea-falt for their Bafis, and are therefore only fo many Kinds of *Aqua regia*; Silver, in *Aqua fortis*, but not in *Aqua regia*, *Spirit of Salt*, *Oil of Vitriol*, or, in fhort, in any but the nitrous Acids; whence it may very properly be faid, that Sea-falt is the true Diffolvent of Gold, and Nitre of Silver. Lead is readily diffolved by the weaker Acids, but not at all by *Aqua regia*, and but difficultly by many of the ftronger; Iron by moft of the acid Salts; and Tin by *Aqua regia*, and not eafily by any other Menftruum, unlefs firft divefted of its Sulphur by Calcination; but *Copper* is to be diffolved by every kind of Salt, and, in fhort, by almoft every thing that ever had in Chemiftry the Name of a Menftruum, and produces, with its different Solvents, an almoft infinite Variety of very beautiful Colours: So that it may indeed have been the Bafis of the Colour of, perhaps, more of the Gems than has yet been imagined

Filings of *Copper* dropt into the Flame of a Lamp, thrown into an horizontal Direction by a Blow-pipe, emit a very beautiful green Flame.

Mixed with three times their Quantity of corrofive Sublimate, and afterwards divefted of the Mercury by Fire, they form, with the remaining Salts, a tranfparent Refin of a beautiful *Hyacinth* Colour, which will melt and burn in the Fire, emitting alfo a fine green Flame.

Expofed to the Fumes of Quickfilver, they become white and fhining like Silver.

Melted with *Zink*, they make an uniform Mafs of a fine gold Colour, as they do Brafs with Calamine.

Held over melted Orpiment, they become not only white but brittle.

And by extreme Violence of Fire, are converted into a hard, denfe, glaffy Matter, of a deep Red; tranfparent, and in fome degree refembling the *Sorane Garnet*.

It has been the general Opinion of the Chemifts, that Solutions of this Metal in Acids were green, and in Alkalies blue, fome, however, have alter'd, from a few Experiments of their own, or perhaps only from what they imagined muft have been the Succefs of Experiments, this general Account, and particularly among fome of the more modern Writers, it has ftood, that *Copper* diffolved in Acids or fix'd Alkalies, affords a green Colour; and in volatile Alkalies, a fine Blue. But you will obferve, by the following Experiments, that thefe Accounts are neither of them to be depended on: And, indeed, whoever has Difquifitions of this kind to attempt, will always find, that it muft be a Knowledge of Nature, and not of Books, that muft afford him what he can depend on, and that Syftems built on any body's Experiments but his own, will be found to ftand on a very infirm Bafis.

What I have been able to learn, by repeated Experiments on this Metal in Menstruums of all kinds, is, that the Solutions of it in different Fluids, cannot be, in regard to Colour, determinately reduced into Method at all; the different Acids having the Properties talk'd of in the Alkalies, of producing different Colours, and even the same Acid being sometimes capable of affording either a green or a blue Solution, according to the different Quantity of the Metal dissolved in it. In Cases of this kind, however, I have every where judged the most perfect Solution the properest to describe the Effect of the Menstruum by. And what I have principally learnt by these Experiments, be pleased to accept the following Account of.

A Solution of *Copper* in Oil of Olives, is of a fine grass Green; in white Wax, of a bluish Green, approaching to the Colour of our *Aqua marine*; and in pure Water, of a dead whitish Green. In regard to these Menstruums it is, however, to be observed, that the express'd vegetable Oils do not dissolve *Copper*, as Oils, but by means of certain other heterogene Particles which they contain; for all express'd vegetable Oils contain in them Water, and a latent acid Salt; of both which, I am pretty certain, they may be wholly divested by Fire, and rendered, by that means, incapable of acting as Menstruums on this Metal; for I have found, that Oil of Olives, after long boiling, has been capable of extracting scarce any Colour at all from *Copper*, and make no doubt but that it might be so perfectly deprived of its Acid, as well as Water, by long boiling with Litharge, or some similar Substance proper to imbibe its Acid, as to have no Power of dissolving this Metal at all. Nor is this latent Acid peculiar to the express'd Oils alone, those procured by Distillation evidently contain it also, as the excellent Dr *Hoffman* has proved, who by grinding the distilled Oils of Lavender and Turpentine with Salt of Tartar, obtained thence a neutral Salt.

Wax, in like manner, dissolves *Copper* no otherwise than by a true, genuine, and pretty sharp Acid, which it evidently contains, and which is easily separated from it by Distillation with a very gentle Heat. And in regard to Water, it may not be improper to observe, that though it is but a poor Dissolvent of Metals with us, yet it may, in the Bowels of the Earth, do Wonders: For we find evidently, that the Power of Water, as a Menstruum, depends, in many Cases, exactly on its Degree of Heat, and as it is capable of the greater Heat, the greater Weight of the Atmosphere it is pressed by, we know not to what Height its Heat and dissolving Power may be raised at great Depths in the Earth.

Of the mineral acid Menstruums, Spirit of Sea-salt, Spirit of Nitre, and *Aqua regia*, all afford green Solutions of *Copper*, but with this Difference, that the Spirit of Salt gives a yellowish Green, the Spirit of Nitre a deep Green, with no Yellowness at all; and the *Aqua regia*, a bright vivid Green, but there is some Admixture of Yellow in it, about in the same measure that it is in some of the Gems which *Pliny* describes by, *Quorum extremus igniculus in flavedinem exeat.* The Solution in Spirit of Nitre is of the true Emerald Colour, and extremely bright and vivid; and each of the others resembles very exactly the Colour of a particular Gem of the same Class; the first of them being perfectly of the Colour of the yellowish green *Prasius*, and the third of the *Smaragdo-prasius*.

These Colours are each of them very beautiful, and that of the Solution in *Aqua regia* is no other than what must be expected, when we know the Colours of the other two, the Spirits of Salt and Nitre being simple Menstruums, and affording a green, and a yellowish green Solution, and the *Aqua regia*, a compound Menstruum, partaking of the Nature of both the others, it must naturally give a Solution of a Colour between both, that is a Green with less Yellow than that of the Spirit of Salt.

But though these three acid Menstruums afford green Solutions of this Metal, it is too hasty a Conclusion to infer from thence, that all the acid Menstruums will therefore do the same; for Solutions of Copper in Oil of Vitriol, Oil of Sulphur, and *Aqua fortis*, are all blue. They are in different Degrees, tho' all nearly approaching to each other, and the deepest of them not darker than that of the common *Turquoises*. These Solutions have also this peculiar Property, that they immediately precipitate their Copper on Iron if immersed in them, and may serve to explain the Effects of those vitriolic Waters which are said to convert Iron into *Copper*. A Piece of Iron Wire dipped into any of these Solutions, and taken almost immediately out again, is seen covered with *Copper* so far as the Menstruum has touched it, and by drawing the Fingers carefully over it, a fine thin Tube of pure *Copper* may be taken off from it. This may serve to shew us of what Kind the Menstruum is which Nature uses to produce the blue Vitriol from *Copper*, which in Solution has the same Effect, and proves that the Ziment or vitriolic Water, so famous for its supposed Virtue, of turning Iron into *Copper*, is no other than a blue Vitriol in a fluid State, because suspended in too large a Quantity of aqueous Matter; perhaps, indeed, containing Particles of many other Kinds, but evidently owing its characteristic Quality, to Particles of *Copper* in a State very nearly resembling that of blue Vitriol, though at present in Solution.

That the natural Colour of Solutions of *Copper* in the vitriolic Acids is blue, is evident from only leaving a Drop of any of them on a Plate of *Copper*, which is presently covered with blue Crystals. And any one a little acquainted with Chemistry will know, that no Difference is to be expected in Solutions made with Oil of Sulphur from those with Oil of Vitriol, for these Acids differ scarce sensibly when both well rectified, and indeed appear, on strict Examination, to be really the same Thing; the same universal mineral Acid, existent every where in the Earth, and sometimes perceiveable by the Senses, in the suffocating Damps of Mines, being the certain Basis of both, as also of a third, that of Alum; and though the different Matter it meets with in Alum, Vitriol, and Sulphur, gives it a different Appearance in the Concrete, yet when freed from that Matter by Chemistry, and rendered as pure as that Art will make it, it appears the same thing whether drawn from one or the other of these Substances.

That Oil of Vitriol, therefore, and Oil of Sulphur, should produce a Solution of *Copper* of the same Colour, is no other than what must naturally be expected. But that *Aqua fortis*, which is a compound Menstruum, and made, though partly from Vitriol, which affords a blue Solution, yet partly also from Nitre, which we have seen before affords a fine green one, should give a simply blue Solution, as it evidently does, without the least Admixture of Green, may seem, at first view, something strange. But here I must observe, that Spirit of Nitre is the Menstruum I hinted at in the Beginning of this Letter, as capable of affording different Colours, from different Quantities of the Metal dissolved in it. And nothing, indeed, is more certain, than that the greenest Solution of *Copper* in Spirit of Nitre, may be turned into a pale Blue, only by adding more and more Filings of the same Metal, up to the proper Quantity for the Change.

These, of all my Experiments on *Copper*, are what have afforded me the greatest Satisfaction in the Subject of the present Enquiry; as they shew, that

Nature is so far from being tied to one single Menstruum for producing the *Sapphirine* Colour from *Copper*, that instead of the Colours of the blue Gems being owing only to the Effects of a single, scarce, and indeed uncertain Menstruum on that Metal, we find they are producible from the Action of others, and those the most common, most abundant, and, indeed, universal Menstruums of the fossile World. We need be no longer at a loss to find where Nature could meet with a sufficient Quantity of a proper Menstruum to extract from *Copper* the Colour necessary for the various blue Gems, when we see, that the universal native fossile Acid, whether in form of Vitriol, Sulphur, or Alum, and unquestionably not less when alone; and even the nitrous, under proper Limitations, are able abundantly to produce it.

Of the vegetable Acids, distilled Vinegar, Lemon-juice, and Spirit of Verdigrease, all give green Solutions of *Copper*; but with this Difference, that the first gives some faint Bluishness with the Green; the second is a pale whitish Green; and the third, the true, pure, and unmixed Green of the *Emerald*.

The fermented vegetable Acids, therefore, have more Effect on this Metal than the native, this is evident from the deeper Colour, and from the much greater Quantity of the Metal separable from Solutions with them, made in the same Proportions: And the Spirit of Verdigrease may very naturally excel both, as it is the strongest vegetable Acid that Art can any way produce; though it is truly no other than a Vinegar abforbed by *Copper*, and afterwards driven from it again by the Force of Fire, little altered, except as rendered more pure. It is remarkable, that *Copper* will thus part with this Acid in its proper and natural Form; whereas no other Metal will, for Iron and Lead, the only other Metals that will admit this Acid, alter it in the Mixture from its original Nature, for it can never be produced from them again in its natural State, but is in both Cafes quite a different thing. When feparated from Lead, it appears in Form of an oily fat Liquor; and from Iron, little other than infipid Water. The Spirit of Verdigreafe is, however, the ftrongeft of all vegetable Acids; and, accordingly, extracts from *Copper* the Colour neareft approaching to that of the Solutions of that Metal in fome of the ftrongeft mineral Acids.

Of the fix'd Alkalies, Salt of Wormwood, Potafhes, and Oil of Tartar *per deliquium*, all afford Solutions of *Copper* of a glorious, deep, celeftial Blue, and no way diftinguifhable from one another, if the Solutions are made in exact Proportions. An *Ærugo*, of a greenifh Colour, is indeed producible on *Copper* by thefe Menftruums, and a fmall Quantity of a fimilar Subftance is fometimes found fwimming on the Surface of thefe very Solutions. But this is not purely the genuine Effect of the Menftruums, but a Change wrought in the Solutions made by them, by Particles of adventitious Salts floating in the Air, and mixing with a fmall Quantity of them. Thefe Changes of Colour in the Solutions of *Copper* from an Admixture of Salts of a different Kind, tho' but in small Quantities, we shall see hereafter in this Letter are very natural and easily producible Effects, and need not wonder at a small Quantity of an *Ærugo* of this kind floating on the Surface of the Menstruum, or affixed to a Plate of Copper wetted with it, and exposed to the Air, tho' the true Solution of *Copper* in the Menstruum is blue; when we consider, that a Solution of the blue Vitriol in a Water impregnated with *Sal Armoniac* is green, notwithstanding that a simple Solution of *Copper* in that Salt is blue, as we shall see hereafter (Such is the endless Variety resulting from Mixtures of Salts as Menstruums) and that the natural *Ærugo* produced on *Copper* by the Salts floating in the Air, is green.

It is not to be wondered at, that the Solutions of *Copper* in the fix'd Alkalies produced from different vegetable Substances, are no way different from one another, since these Bodies act in these Solutions, not as the peculiar Salts of this or that Plant, but as a Body made, not by any Operation of Nature, but by the Effect of Fire, which has strongly united the essential Salt, the Earth, and some small Portion of the Oil of the Vegetable they have been prepared from. For all these fix'd Alkalies of Plants may be resolved into a bitter saline Substance, a stronger fix'd Alkali, and a pure simple Earth, and in the Operation there will a small Quantity of an oily Matter always be discovered.

Of the volatile Alkalies, Spirit of *Sal Armoniac*, Spirit of Urine, and Spirit of Hartshorn, all afford

Solutions of *Copper* of the moſt beautiful and vivid celeſtial Blue, this is of different Degrees, according to the different Quantity of the Metal diſſolved; but in equal Proportions, and with the Spirits of equal Strength, the Colour is exactly the ſame in them all. The volatile Alkalies have in their Operations on this Metal, therefore, a great Analogy to the fix'd. Theſe Menſtruums conſiſt only of a very fine, ſubtle, volatile, alkaline Salt, ſuſpended in a ſmall Quantity of Water, which has no Share in extracting this glorious Colour; for the dry volatile Salts of the ſame Subſtances, mixed with Copper Filings, and corked up in a Vial together, acquire, in a Day or two, the very ſame Colour.

Of the neutral Salts, a Solution of *Copper* with crude *Sal Armoniac*, is of a glorious Blue, with native *Borax*, of a fine deep Green; and with Sea-ſalt, of a pale whitiſh Green: Of theſe, the *Sal Armoniac* diſſolves it the ſooneſt, the Sea ſalt takes more time, and the *Borax* is ſloweſt of all. The reſt of the Solutions alſo mentioned here, require different Time and different Methods to produce them; the Spirit of Nitre diſſolves the Metal almoſt inſtantaneouſly, *Aqua fortis* is nearly as quick in its Operation, and *Aqua regia* requires only a little Time, but of the others, ſome require long and tedious Proceſſes, and others act beſt, or perhaps only, by Vapour; and one of theſe Proceſſes ſhews, that where Mr *Boyle* ſays, he knew a Menſtruum which by its Vapour would diſſolve a certain Metal, though it would ſcarce work on it at all in Subſtance; he is only talking of Copper and Vinegar. *Sal Armoniac,* it is to be also obferved, affords us another Inftance whence Nature may be fupplied with a Menftruum for giving a blue Solution of *Copper,* fince, tho' the *Sal Armoniac* common among us now is factitious, there is no queftion but that there is, and ever has been, a true native *Sal Armoniac*; and there needs no more than *Copper* diffolved in Water impregnated with it, to give the different Blues of all the deepeft *Sapphires* in the World; it being moft eafy to procure a Solution of *Copper* of any degree of blue, only from a Solution of this Salt in Water, digefted for a few Days on Filings of that Metal.

The Colours producible from Salt and Borax may eafily be imagined to be alfo plentiful enough, fince the Salt of Salt-fprings and *Sal Gem* are evidently the fame with Sea falt in all refpects, and are abundant every where in the Earth; and native Borax is found to be plentiful enough in fome Parts of the World, and perhaps is in many others alfo, where it has not been yet difcovered

Thefe, Sir, are a few of the many Experiments the Enquiry after what Menftruum Nature has ufed to impart, by the Affiftance of *Copper,* the Blue Colour to the *Sapphire, Turquoife,* and other blue Gems, has led me into. A great many more might have been mentioned, and much more faid on the Action of thefe; but as thefe are felected, fo as to give Proofs of the Action of two or three Menftruums of every Kind, and what regards the End proposed, every where mentioned in the Observations on them, more would have been unnecessary. From what is observed, however, it is easy to infer, that more of the Gems than barely those I have occasion to treat of here, may owe their Colour to this Metal; and even more, in reality may, than I have yet given Hints for the conjecturing at, for what I have hitherto described, are only the Effects of the simple Menstruums which are here described. But Nature, we should remember, may also use compound ones: And what an almost infinite Variety of Colourings may arise from such Mixtures it is scarce to be conceived; for not only different Colours may be produced from the Effects of different Menstruums combined, in order to work on the Metal, but even the same Colour already procured, may be almost infinitely varied from the Action of new Menstruums upon it. Thus a Solution of *Copper* in any of the before mentioned Acids, so weak as to leave the Menstruum colourless like Water, may in an Instant, by the Affusion of a few Drops of Oil of Tartar *per deliquium*, be converted into a glorious Blue, or by a like Quantity of Spirit of Nitre, into a beautiful Green. Nay, when by this means made Blue, may be yet changed into green by a larger Quantity of the Acid. And even when thus made green, again converted into its former blue, by a yet larger quantity of the Alkali.

The blue Tinctures of *Copper* made in the fix'd Alkalies, may also be divested of their Colour, and rendered colourless and pellucid like Water, by Acids, if the Proportions be carefully regarded: The blue Liquor here is made colourless, as the colourless Liquor was before made blue; and the pellucid Liquid thus produced, will exhibit all the Phænomena before described in that originally colourless. To this it may be added, that even the strong blue and green Solutions are easily changed from blue to green, and from green to blue, in the same Manner. But I shall have Opportunity to speak of these Changes more at large in another Place; as I intend, with your Permission, to shew before the ROYAL SOCIETY, these and some other Experiments on the original Rise, Destruction, Reproduction, and Changes, of the Colours of the Solutions of this Metal.

The great Thing that I have aimed to prove by these Experiments, is however, I presume, by this time, rendered clear and incontestable; That Nature is not tied to one only Menstruum for the producing Blue from Copper, and that but a very scarce and uncertain one. Since it is evident, that the Bodies necessary to give it are many, and those, many of them common and every where abundant. That the common and universal mineral Acid, so abundant every where in all the Kinds of *Pyrites*, the Acid of Sulphur, Vitriol, or Alum; which are, I have said, the same with the former, and with each other, in different Combinations, can do it. And even no better a Menstruum than common Water passing over a Quantity of native *Sal Armoniac*, is able to produce from *Copper*, all the different Degrees of Blue, from that of the palest to that of the deepest Oriental *Sapphires*.

I am, with the greatest Respect,

SIR,

Broad-way, Westminster,
June 19, 1746

Your most Obedient

Humble Servant,

JOHN HILL.

GREEK INDEX.

A

Ἀδάμας   Pag. 46
Αἰγύπτι⟨ος⟩ Κυανός   130
Αἰγύπτῳ, Ἄνθρακες ἐκ   90
Αἱματίτις   96
————— Ξανθὴ καλευμένη   96
Ἄκαυστοι λίθοι τινές   12
Ἄκαυστον γένος λίθων   40
Ἀλόνη   108
Ἀλαβαςρίτης   22
————— καλέμεν⟨ος⟩ Ὄνυξ, n.   23
Ἀμέθυσον   80
————— οἰνωπὸν τῇ χρόᾳ   84
Ἀνθράκιον   80
————— ἐκ Ἀρκαδίας   88
Ἄνθραξ   26, 40
————— ἐκ Καρχηδόνος   44
————— ἐκ Μασσιλίας   ibid.
————— περὶ Μίλητον   ibid.
————— Κορίνθι⟨ος⟩   88
————— Τροιζήνι⟨ος⟩   ibid.
Ἄνθρακες περιττοὶ σπάνιοι   ibid.
————— ἐκ Αἰγύπτῳ   90
————— ἐκ Συήνης   ibid.
————— ἐκ Ψηφοῦ   ibid.
Ἄνθραξ γηώδης   38
Ἀπολίθωσις   118
Ἀραβικὸς λίθ⟨ος⟩   50
Ἄργυρον κινῶν   138

(192)

Ἀρμενίας, λίθοι ἐξ	108
Ἀρρενικὸν	102
Ἀσίας, λίθοι ἐξ	142
Ἀςὴρ	148
Ἄτηκτοι λίθοι	12
Ἀχάτης	86

B

Βακτριανῆς, Σμάραγδοι ἐκ	97
—— ὁ μεγάλοι	ibid
Βίναις, λίθοι περὶ	37

Γ

Γῆ	2
Γῆς ἰδιώτεραι διαφοραὶ	114
Γῆ Λημνία, η	126
— Κιμωλία	142
— Μηλίας	ibid
— Σαμία	ibid
— Τυμφαϊκὴ	ibid
Γλυπτοὶ λίθοι	18
Γύψος	142, 150
—— ἐν Θυρέοις	152
—— ἐν Κύπρῳ	152
—— ἐν Συρίᾳ	150, 156
—— ἐν Φοινίκῃ	ibid.
—— ἔμπυρός ἐστι	156
—— ἰσχύς ἐστι	ibid.
Γύψου χρῶν⟨⟩ πρὸς τὰ οἰκοδομήματα	154
Γύψου χρῆσις πυρώδης	158

Δ

Διαφοραὶ τῶν λίθων	20
Δυνάμεις τῶν λίθων	12

E

Ἐλέφας ὄρυκτὸς	94
—— ποικίλ⟨⟩ μέλανι	ibid·
Ἐφέσου, Κιννάβαρι ἐκ	136
—— εὕρημα Καλλίου	138

Ἤλεκτρον

Η

Ἤλεκτρον	78
——— ὀρυκτὸν περὶ Λιγυστικὴν	ibid.
——— αὐτοῦ ἕλκειν δύναμις	ibid.
Ἡράκλεια λίθος	16

Θ

Θηβαϊκὸς λίθος	20
Θραυςοὶ λίθοι	32
Θυρίοις; Γύψος ἐν	152

Ι

Ἴασπις	58
——— ἐν Κύπρῳ	90
Ἰβηρίαν περὶ, Κιννάβαρι	134
Ἰδιότητες ἐν τοῖς λίθοις	12
Ἰὸς	134

Κ

Κάλαμος Ἰνδικὸς ἀπολιθωμένος	100
Καρχηδόνιος, Ἄνθραξ	44
Καυςοὶ λίθοι	12
Κεραμὸς	30
Κιλικίαν, γῆ περὶ	118
——— ταύτῃ ἀλείφουσι τὰς ἀμπέλους	ibid.
Κιμωλία γῆ	142
Κιννάβαρι	134
——— αὐτοφυὲς	ibid.
——— κατ' ἐργασίαν	ibid.
——— αὐτοφυὲς περὶ Ἰβηρίαν	ibid.
——— κατ' ἐργασίαν ἐξ Ἐφέσου	136
——— ἔςιν ἄμμος	ibid.
Κίσηρις	38
——— ἐκ κατακαύσεως	48
——— ἐξ ἀφροῦ θαλάσσης	ibid.
——— περὶ τὰς κρατῆρας	50
——— ἐκ τοῦ Ἀραβικοῦ λίθου	ibid.
——— σμηρικολάτη ἐκ θαλάσσης	56
——— μυλώδης	ibid.

O   Κίσηρις

Κίσηρις ἐν Νισύρῳ	52
——— ἐν Μήλῳ	38, 54
——— ἐν Σικελίᾳ	56
Κιχώριον, η	147
Κεράμιον	96
——— φύεϑ ἐν τῇ θαλάτῃ	ibid
Κορίνθι@ Ἄνθραξ	88
Κρύσαλλ@	80
Κυανός	82, 102
——— Αἰγύπτι@	130
——— ἄῤῥην ἡ θῆλυς	82
——— μελάντερ@ ὁ ἄῤῥην	ibid.
——— αὐτοφυὴς	100
——— ἔχων χρυσόκολλαν	102
——— ἐλάχις@	122
——— Κύπρι@	130
——— Σκύθης	ibid
——— ὁ Αἰανὸς	ibid
Κυανᾶ γλύη τερα	ibid
Κύπειρ@ Κυκνὸς	ibid.
Κύπρῳ ἐν, Σμάραγδ@	90
——— Ἴασπις	ibid
Κυτὸ Ἄργυρον	138
——— ἐκ Κιννάβαρι	ibid.

Λ

Λαμψάκου λίθ@	86
Λημνία γῆ	126
Λίθοι ἄτιμοι	12
——— τίμιοι	ibid
——— γλυπτοί	18
——— πιστοί	ibid
——— πριστοί	ibid.
——— θραυστοί	32
——— περὶ Βίνας	ibid
——— τικτοι	16
Λίθ@ Ἀραβικὸς	50
——— ἐν Ταινάροιδι	38

Λίθος ἐν Ἐρινεάδι	38
—— ἄνθραξι ὅμοια	102
—— βασανίζουσα τ̀ χρυσόν	110
—— δ̇ίρισπε] ἐν Τμώλῳ	112
—— Ἡράκλεια	16
—— Λυδή	ibid.
—— ΛιπαραῖΘ·	36
—— Πάριθ·	20
—— Πεντελικός	ibid.
—— ΧῖΘ·	ibid.
—— Θηβαῖος	ibid.
—— ὁ σίδηρον ἄγουσα	78
—— —— σπανία	ibid.
Λίθων χρῶ· ἄκαυςον	40
—— διαφοραί	20
—— μεταλλουργῶν φύσεις	100
ΛιπαρεῖΘ· λίθΘ·	36
Λυγκούριον	72
—— ἕλκει ὥσπερ τὸ ἠλ. ἤγουν	74
—— ἄρρεν κ̀ θῆλυ	82
Λυδή	16

M

Μαγνῆτις λίθΘ·	104
Μαργαρῖτις	92
—— ἐν ὀστρείῳ τινί	ibid.
—— ἐν τ̀ πίνναις	ibid.
Μάρμαρθ·	28
Μασσαλίας ἐκ, ἄνθραξ	44
Μηλίας γῆ	142
Μυλῶν, σίδηρος	54
Μιλήτου πὲ, ἄνθραξ	44
ΜίλΘ·	102, 122, 124
—— αὐτόματΘ·	130
—— τεχνική	ibid.
—— βελτίστη ἐν Κέᾳ	124
—— ἐν τ̀ μετάλλων	ibid.
—— Λημνία	126

Μίλτ۞ Σινοπική	126
——— ἔςιν Καππαδοκικὴ	ibid
Μυλίαι	26
Μυλώδης κίοσηεις	56

Ν

Νισύρῳ ἐν, κίοσηεις	52

Ξ

Ξάνθη	96

Ο

Ὀβελισκὸς ἐκ τετ]άρων Σμαράγδων	64
Ὄμφαξ	80
Ὄνυξ	84
Ὀρχομενῶ ἐξ, ἀνθεμίον	88
Ὀψιανὸς λίθ۞, π.	24

Π

Παρί۞ λίθ۞	20
Πεντελικὸς λίθ۞	ibid
Πῆξις ἀπὸ θερμῦ	10
——— ἀπὸ ψυχρῦ	ibid.
Περσίτης	96
——— ἰώδης τῇ χρόᾳ	ibid.
Περσοὶ λίθοι	18
Πυρομάχοι	26
Πῶρ۞	22

Σ

Σαμία γῆ	142
Σαιδαράκη	102
Σάπφειρ۞	26
——— χρυσόπας۞	58
Σάρδιον	26, 82
Σαρκόφαγ۞, π.	14
Σιδήρεον τῶνδε λίθων ἐχ ἅπ]ε].	18
Σικελία ἐν, κίοσηεις	56
Σινοπικὴ γῆ	126
——— αὐτῆς γένη τρία	ibid.
——— ἐρυθρά	ibid.
——— ἐκλακτ۞	128

Σινοπικὴ αὐτάρκη	128
——— ἐκ τ̃ ὄχεϑς καΙακαιομρύης	ibid.
——— εὕρημα Κυδίκ	ibid.
Σίφνι۞ λίθ۞	106
Σκαπίησυλης λίθ۞	40
Σκύθης Κυανὸς	130
Σμάρᾳγδ۞	14, 26, 62
——— ἐν Κύπρῳ	90
——— ἐκ τ̃ Βακιερανῆς	92
——— ϖειτὴ τῇ δυνάμ৭	72
——— πρὸς τὰ ὄμμαΙα ἀγαθὴ	62
——— ἐκ τ̃ Ἰάαπιδ۞	70
——— Τανὸς ιαλέμρυ۞	64
——— ἐξομοιοῦται τ̃ χρόαν ὑδαΙ۞ ἑαυτῇ	62
——— ἡ μεγάλη	ibid.
Σμίϱις, n.	108
Σπιλ۞, n.	34
Σπίν۞	ibid
Σιλήνης, Ἄνθϱακες ἐν	90
Σφϱαγὶς, n.	25
Σφϱαγίδιον, n.	ibid.

Τ

Τανὸς	64
Τέlεφάδι, λίθοι ἐν	38
Τηκὶοι λίθοι	12
Τικίοὶ λίθοι	16
Τμώλῳ, λίθοι ἐν	112
Τυμφαικὴ γῆ	142
Τορευτοὶ λίθοι	18
Τροιζήνι۞ Ἄνθϱαξ	85

Υ

Ὑαλοειδὴς	80
Ὕδωρ	2
Ὕλιτις	116
——— ὕελ۞ ἐκ	ibid.
——— χάλικι μιγνυμένη	118
Ὕελ۞	116

Φ

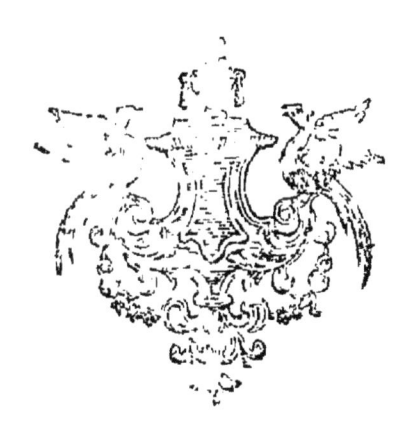

Φάελδι ἐν, Μηλιὰς γῆ	116
Φύσεις ἰδιώτεραι γῆς	4

Χ

Χερνίτης	22
Χῖος λίθος	20
Χρυσοκόλλα	70, 102
Χρυσόπας Σάπφειρος	58

Ψ

Ψευδὴς Σμάραγδος	66
—— περὶ Κύπρον	68
—— ἐν τῇ νήσῳ ὑπὸ λαμβάνει χαλκηδόνι	ibid.
Ψῆβα, Ἄνθρακες ἐκ	90
Ψιμύθιον	132

Ω

Ὤχρα	102, 122, 124

THE GENERAL INDEX.

N. B. *The Letter n refers to the Notes.*

A

ACID Salt in expressed Oils,	Page 178
in distilled Oils,	ibid.
ADAMAS Cyprius, n	110
ÆGYPTIAN Carbuncles,	91
ÆTITES Lapis,	17
AFFLUX, Fossils form'd by it,	7
AGAIF,	87
what, and whence brought, n	86
Leonine, n	87
Its various Kinds, n	86
ALABANDINE, n	45
ALABASTER,	23
Gypsum made from it, n.	148
AMANDINE, n.	46
AMBER,	79
a native Fossil,	ibid
erroneous Opinions about it, n.	78
AMETHYST,	81
owes its Colour to Iron, n	82
loses its Colour in the Fire, n.	ibid.
AMPELITES Lapis, n	36
AQUILINUS Lapis, n.	17
ARABICUS Lapis,	51
ARMENIA, Stones thence to cut others with,	109

(200)

ARMENUS *Lapis*,   103
       Ægyptian,   131
       Scythian,   ibid
       Cyprian,   ibid.
       fictitious   ibid
ASIA, stony Masses thence,   143
ASPHALTUM, n   35
ASSIUS *Lapis*, n   14
ASTER, a kind of *Samian* Earth,   149
ATTRACTION the Cause of Cohesion of Fossils,   10

B

BACTRIANA, Emeralds found there   92
BALASS Ruby, n   46
BASANITES *Lapis*, n.   111
BERGBLAU, n   102
BELEMNITES, n.   74
BENA, bituminous Stones found there,   33
BERYLLUS *Oleaginus* of *Pliny*, n.   81
BITUMEN *Judaicum*, n   35
BLOODSTONE, or *Hæmatites*,   97
——————— or *Heliotropes*, n   58
BOLES, what, n.   116
BRICKS,   117
BROCATELLO of the *Italians*, n   22

C

CÆRULEUM *nativum*,   103
       fictitious, of *Egypt*,   131
CALAMUS *Indicus* petrified   101
CALLAIS, n.   95
CALLIMUS of the Eagle stone, how form'd, n.   19
CALLIAS, Inventer of a factitious Cinnabar,   139
CALX *nativa*, n   148
CANNEL Coal, n   36
CAPPADOCIA, Reddle dug there   125
       the *Rubrica Sinopica* dug there,   137
CARBUNCLE,   27, 43, 45, 81
       Ægyptian,   91

Carthaginian,	91
Corinthian,	89
Massilian,	91
of *Orchomenus*,	89
of *Tsebos*,	91
of *Syene*,	ibid.
Træzenian,	89
CARNELIAN,	27, 56, 59, 83, ----
Male and Female	83
CARTHAGE, Carbuncles had thence,	45
Emeralds found there	69
CEA, fine Reddle thence	125
CERACHATES, n.	86
CERUSE, how made,	183
CHALKS, what, n	116
CHERT, a kind of Flint, n.	30
CHERNITIS,	23
CHIAN Marble,	21
CHOLUS, a kind of Emerald, n.	65
CHRYSITIS *Lapis*, n	111
CHRYSOCOLLA,	71, 113
of the Antients, what, n.	70
CHRYSOPRASUS, n.	96
CILICIAN Earth,	119
CIMOLIAN Earth,	143
of the Antients, what, n	144
CINNABAR,	135
native,	ibid.
what, and where found, n	136
found in *Spain*,	137
factitious,	135
when first found out	139
from *Ephesus*,	137
procured from a red Sand,	ibid.
first found by *Callias*,	139
Dragons-blood so called,	136
CLAYS, what, n.	116
COAL,	39
COHESION of Fossils, the Cause of it, n.	31
COLCHIS, Cinnabar found there,	137
COLD, Concretion of some Fossils owing to it,	11

COPPER, soluble in all Salts, 176
    dissolved in *Aqua fortis*, 180
        in *Aqua regia*, 179
        with Borax, 186
        in distilled Vinegar, 183
        in Juice of Lemons, ibid
        in Oil of Vitriol, 180
        in Oil of Sulphur, ibid
        in Oil of Tartar 184
        in Oil of Olives 178
        with Pot-ashes 184
            Salt of Wormwood, ibid.
            Sal Ammoniac, 186
            Sea-Salt, ibid.
        in Spirit of *Sal Ammoniac*, 185
        in Spirit of Hartshorn, ibid.
        in Spirit of Urine, ibid.
        in Spirit of Nitre, 179, 182
        in Spirit of Salt, ibid
        in Spirit of Verdigrease 183
        in Water, 178
        in Wax, ibid.
CORAL, 97
    a Vegetable 98, 99
COTHON, Emeralds found there, n. 68
COTICULA, n. 109
CRYSTAL, 81
CRYSTALLINE Balls echinated, n ibid
        concave, n. ibid
CYANUS, 83
    Male and Female, ibid.
    what and whence, n 84
CYPRIAN Diamonds, what, n. 110
CYPRUS, *Gypsum* thence, 151
    Emeralds found there, 69

D

DEAN, Forest of, Reddle thence, n. 123
DENDRACHATES, n. 86
DIAMOND, 47

E

EAGLE Stone, n.	17
EARTH, the original Structure of it, n.	7
Structure of it after the Deluge,	8
EARTH, what,	113
its various Kinds, n.	116
how coloured, n.	142
vitrifiable,	117
Cilician, used to Vines,	119
coloured Kinds used by Painters,	121
Cimolian	143
of the Antients, what, n.	144
of the Moderns, what,	145
Lemnian, n.	126
Melian,	143
of the Antients, what, n.	142
Samian,	149
not used by Painters,	145
of the Antients, what, n.	ibid.
how dug,	147
called *After*,	149
called *Collyrion*, n.	147
Tymphaican,	143
called *Gypsum*,	149
the Basis of Stones,	3
petrifying,	119
ELATITIS, a kind of Blood-stone, n.	97
EMERALD,	27, 61, ----
its History, n.	61, 62, 63, 64
Oriental, n.	63
European, n.	62
Scythian, n.	64
Persian, n.	ibid.
Ægyptian, n.	ibid.
from *Cyprus*,	91
Bactriana, how found,	92
seeming produced from the *Jasper*,	73
from Chrysocolla,	71
of enormous Size in *Egypt*,	65
called *Tanus*,	ibid.
Bastard, where found,	69

EMERALD strikes a Green through Water,	15, 63
good for the Eyes,	63
other medicinal Virtues of it,	72
EMERY, known to the Antients, n.	108
ERINEAS, Stone found there	39

F

FIRE, how it occasions Fluidity, n	31
Stones not hurt by it,	41
why some Stones not hurt by it,	49
FLINTS, Formation of them, n	18
used in making Glass,	119
FORMATION, original, of Fossils, n.	6
FOSSILS, all fusible, n	114
FUSION, Humidity necessary to it,	31
General Cause of it, n.	32

G

GAGATES, n.	35
GARNET, n.	46
Sorane, n.	ibid
GEMS, coloured by metalline Particles, n	43
Difficulty of methodizing them, n.	42
Male and Female,	83
GEODES, or bastard Eagle-stone, n	19
GLASS,	117
of the Moderns, how made, n.	118
of the Antients, how made,	119
blue, what,	176
GOLD, Stone that trys it,	111
GYPSUM,	151
the Antients had many Kinds, n.	148
of *Cyprus*,	151
of *Phœnicia*,	ibid.
of *Thuria*,	153
of *Syria*,	151
of *Tymphæa*,	153
made of different Stones, n.	151
of Stones like Alabaster,	153
used in Buildings,	155
how prepared for Use,	ibid.

used about Cloaths,	157
of *Syria*, how made,	ibid.
its Nature owing to Fire,	159
Tymphaican Earth so called,	149
GYPSINUM *Metallum*, what, n.	152

H

HÆMACHATES, n.	86
HÆMATITES *Lapis*,	97
HEAT, Concretion of some Fossils owing to it,	11
HELIOTROPE, n.	58
HERACLIAN Stone,	17, 111
HYACINTH, n.	47
La Bella, n.	77
HYALOIDES,	81
the *Astrios* of *Pliny*, n.	80

J

JASPACHATES, n.	86
JASPER,	59
from *Cyprus*,	91
the Matrix of the *Prasius*, n.	71
sometimes emulates the *Prasius*, n.	ibid.
JET, n.	35
IRIS, n	81
IVORY, fossile,	95
altered more or less in the Earth, n.	94
Turquoise of this kind, n	ibid.

K

KALI, Salt of it used in Glass-making, n	117

L

LAMPSACUS, Stone found there,	87
LAPIS *Armenus*,	103
yields four Colours,	133
factitious,	131
Ægyptian,	ibid.
Scythian,	ibid.
Cyprian,	ibid.

LAPIS *Specularis*, *Gypsum* made of it, n.	148
LEMNIAN Earth, n.	126
Reddle,	127
LEUCACHATES, n	86
LIPARA Stone,	37
LITHANTHRAX, n.	40
LOADSTONE, n.	79
LOAMS, what, n.	117
LYDIAN Stone,	17, 111
where found,	113
Tryal by it how made,	ibid
Difference in the Sides,	ibid
Tries best in cold Weather,	115
LYNCURIUS *Lapis*,	73, 75, 77
of the Antients, what, n	74, 75
Male and Female,	83

M

MAGNET Gem,	105
of the Antients, what, n	100
MARLES, what, n	116
MARBLE, not fufible in the Fire,	29
Parian,	21
Pentelican,	ibid
Chian,	ibid
Theban,	ibid.
MASSILIA, Carbuncles thence,	45, 91
MELIAN Earth,	143
of the Antients, what, n	142
white, not yellow, n	ibid.
MELOS, Pumices found there,	55
MENDIP Hills, Ochre thence, n	122
MEROPE, an Island, the fame with *Siphnas*, n.	106
MESALUM *Gypsum*, what, n	152
MILETIAN Carbuncle,	45
MILTOS of the Greeks, what, n.	123
MINIUM, n	123, 135
MOCHO Stones, n	86
MOLARIS *Lapis*,	27
a kind of *Pyrites*, n.	29
MOULD vegetable, n.	115
MUNDICK, n.	30

(207)

N

NEPHRITICUS *Lapis*, n.	96
NISUROS, Pumices found there,	53

O

OBSIDIANUS *Lapis*, n.	24
OCHRE,	103
what, n.	116
Yellow, two Kinds, n	122
OMPHAX,	81
the *Beryllus Oleaginus* of *Pliny*, n.	ibid.
ONEAGH, petrifying Lake there, n.	119
ONYCHITES *Marmor*, n	22
ONYX,	85
what, and whence brought, n	85
Alabaster so called, n.	84
ORCHOMENUS, Carbuncle thence,	89
ORMUZ, Gulph of, red Earth thence, n.	123
ORPIMENT,	103, 121
what, and whence brought, n	104
becomes red in burning,	ibid
OSTRACITES, Gems polished with it,	109

P

PARIAN Marble,	21
PEARL,	93
what, and whence brought, n.	92, 93
PEBBLES, how formed, n	18
PERCOLATION, Fossils formed by it,	7
PENTELICAN Marble,	21
PETRIFYING Earths,	119
Stone,	15
PHOENICIAN Gypsum,	151
PHOENICIANS pay their Tribute in *Lapis Armenus*,	133
PHARIS, *Melian* Earth of that Place,	147
PINNA *Marina*, Pearl in it,	93
PISSASPHALTOS, n	35
PORUS, a Marble so called,	23
PRASIUS,	97
what, and whence brought, n.	96

PRINCIPLES of mixed Bodies, 4
PSEBOS, Carbuncles thence, 91
PSEUDO-*Adamantes*, 81
    Smaragdus, 67
PUMICE, 49
  made by Fire, ibid.
    from the Froth of the Sea, ibid.
      by burning the *Lapis Arabicus*, 51
  different Kinds formed different Ways, 53
  in the Openings of the burning Mountains, 51
  of *Nisuros*, 53
  of *Melos*, 55
  black, of the *Sicilian* Shores, 57
  only a Cinder made by burning, n. 49
  different Stones called by this Name, n. 52
  of *Nisuros*, was probably a *Pyrites*, n. 53
PYRITÆ, 27
  what they contain, n 29
PYRRHOPOEICLUS of *Pliny*, n. 22

Q

QUALITIES, different of Fossils, whence, 9
QUICKSILVER, 139
  Ways of extracting it from Cinnabar, n. 138
  found pure in the Earth, n. 140
  Errors of the Antients about it, n 141

R

REDDLE, 103
  of two Kinds, 131
  of several Kinds, n. 123
  that of the Pits preferred, 125
  contains Iron, n 124
  Lemnian, 127
  Sinopic, ibid
    what, and whence, n. 128
    a native *Crocus Martis*, n. 127
ROCK Ruby, n 46
ROT *gulden Ertz*, n. 101
RUBACELLE, n. 46

RUBY, true, n. 46
    Balass, n ibid.
    Spinell, n. ibid.

S

SALTS, lixivial, what, 185
SALT acid in expressed Oils, 178
    in distilled Oils, ibid.
SAMIAN Earth, 143
    not used by Painters, 145
    of the Antients, what, ibid.
    how dug, 147
    called *Aster*, 149
    called *Collyrion*, 147
SAMOS, Pits there, ibid.
SAND, what, n. 115
SANDARACH, 103, 121
SANDASIRUM, n 47
SARCOPHAGUS *Lapis*, n. 14
SAPPHIRE, 27, 59, 95
    of the Antients, what, n. 59
    of the Moderns, n. 60
    counterfeit, how made, 170
SARDACHATES, n 86
SCAPILSYLÆ, Stones found there, 41
SICILIAN Pumices, 57
SIL *Atticum*, what, n. 135
SINOPIC Earth, 127
    dug in *Cappadocia*, ibid
    three Kinds of it, ibid.
    found in *America*, n. 129
    a Kind of it made of Ochre, ibid
SINOPIS, a common Name for red Earths, n 130
SIPHNUS, Stone found there, 107
SMARAGDO *Prasus*, n. 96
SMIRIS, n 108
SOAP Rock, n 145
SOLIDITY of Fossils, Cause of it, n 31
SPAIN, Native Cinnabar found there, 137
SPHRAGIS, n 126
SPINELL Ruby, n. 46

P

SPINUS, 35
SPARS, n. 26
    formed by Percolation and Afflux, ibid
    their natural Colour white, n 27
    assume their Shape from Metals, n. ibid.
    coloured by Metals, n 28
    not fusible in the Fire, ibid
STALAGMITÆ, n 9
STALACTITÆ, n. ibid.
STEATITES, n 145
STONE attracting Iron, 79
STONES containing Gold and Silver, 101
    resembling Carbuncles, but heavier, 103
    which bring forth Young, 17
    the different Kinds, whence, 13
    different fit for different Works, 19
    some not to be cut by Iron, 105
        but by other Stones, 107
    fusible, 27
SYENE, Carbuncles thence, 91
SYENITES of *Pliny*, n 22
SYRIA, *Gypsum* thence, 151

T

TANUS, a Kind of Emerald, 65
    a large one in *Tyre*, ibid.
TERRA *Lemnia*, n. 126
    Sinopica, 127
        what, and whence, n. 128
    Cimolia, 143
    Melia, ibid
    Samia, 145
    Tymphaica, 143
TERRE *Verte*, n. 142
TETRAS, Stones found there, 39
THEBAN Marble, 21
THRACIUS *Lapis*, n 32
TOPAZ, n 44
TOPHUS, 23
    the same with the *Topfstein* of the *Germans*, ibid
TROEZENIAN Carbuncle, 89

TURQUOISE, n.	94
coloured by Copper, n.	94, 163
rough,	94, 171
TYMPHAICAN Earth,	143
called *Gypsum*,	149

V

VEGETABLE Mould, what, n.	115
UELITIS,	119
VERD' *Azur*, n.	102
VERDELLO, n.	111
VERDIGREASE, how made,	135
VINEGAR, a Solvent of Copper,	183
VIRTUES of the Gems enquired into, n.	73
UNIONES, n.	93

W

WATER, considered as a Menstruum,	179
Copper dissolved in it,	178
the Basis of Metals,	3
WATERS petrifying, n.	120
WAX, a Solvent of Copper,	178
by what Means,	179
WHERN, a kind of Flint, n.	30
WHETSTONES,	109
WOOD petrified, n.	120

X

XANTHUS, a kind of Hæmatites,	97

Y

YELLOW Ochres,	122

Z

ZAFFER, native, whether existent,	166
common, how made,	ibid.
blue Gems supposed coloured by it,	164
why supposed so,	165
the Arguments considered,	168, 169, 170
ZARNICH *Asfar*, n.	104
Ahmer, n.	ibid.
ZIMENT,	181

FINIS.

BOOKS printed for C. DAVIS.

I. *Elements* of the Art of *Aſſaying Metals*, in two Parts; the firſt containing the *Theory*, the ſecond the *Practice* of the ſaid *Art*. The whole deduced from the true Properties and Nature of *Foſſils*, confirmed by the moſt accurate and unqueſtionable Experiments, explained in a natural Order, and with the utmoſt Clearneſs. By *John Andrew Cramer*, M.D. Tranſlated from the *Latin*, and illuſtrated with *Copper Plates*. To which are added ſeveral *Notes* and *Obſervations*, not in the Original, particularly uſeful to the *Engliſh* Reader. With an Appendix, containing a Liſt of the chief *Authors*, that have been publiſhed in *Engliſh*, upon *Minerals* and *Metals*. 8vo.

II. *The compleat Mineral Laws of Derbyſhire*, taken from the Originals, 1. The *High Peak Laws*, with their Cuſtoms. 2. *Stony Middleton* and *Eame*, with a new Article made, 1733. 3. The Laws of the Manor of *Aſhforth i'th' Water*. 4. The *Low Peak Articles*, with their Laws and Cuſtoms. 5. The Cuſtoms and Laws of the Liberty of *Litton*. 6. The Laws of the Lordſhip of *Tidſwell*. And all their Bills of Plaint, Cuſtoms, Croſs Bills, Arreſts, Plaintiff's Caſe, or Brief; with all other Forms neceſſary for all Miners and Maintainers of Mines within each *Manour*, *Lordſhip*, or *Wapentake*.

> *Quid dulcius Hominum Generi, à Natura datum eſt, quam jus cuique liberi.*

III. The *Natural*, *Experimental*, and *Medicinal* Hiſtory, of the *Mineral Waters* of *Derbyſhire*, *Lincolnſhire*, and *Yorkſhire*, particularly thoſe of *Scarborough*, wherein they are carefully examined and compared, their Contents diſcovered and divided, their Uſes ſhewn and explained, and an Account given of their Diſcovery and Alterations. Together with the Natural Hiſtory of the *Earths*, *Minerals*, and *Foſſils*, through which the chief of them paſs, the groundleſs Theories and falſe Opinions of former Writers are expoſed, and their Reaſonings demonſtrated to be injudicious and inconcluſive. To which are added large marginal Notes, containing a methodical Abſtract of all the Treatiſes hitherto publiſhed on theſe *Waters*, with many Obſervations and Experiments, as alſo four *Copper Plates*, repreſenting the Cryſtals of the Salts of Thirty four of thoſe Waters. By *Thomas Short*, M.D. of *Sheffield*. In two Volumes Quarto.

IV. *The Hiſtory and Antiquities of Harwich and Dover court*, *Typographical*, *Dynaſtical*, and *Political*. Firſt collected by *Silas Taylor*, alias *Domville*, Gent. Keeper of the King's Stores there; and now much enlarged in all its Parts; with Notes and Obſervations relating to Natural Hiſtory. Illuſtrated with *Copper Plates* repreſenting the *Cliff* itſelf, the *Foſſils* contained therein, and other principal Things, by *Samuel Dale*.